RUNNING THAT DOESN'T SUCK

HOW TO LOVE RUNNING
(EVEN IF YOU THINK YOU HATE IT)

LISA JHUNG

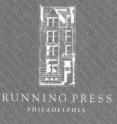

RUNNING PRESS
PHILADELPHIA

Running Press
Hachette Book Group
1290 Avenue of the Americas, New York, NY 10104
www.runningpress.com
@Running_Press

Printed in the United States

First Edition: July 2019

Published by Running Press, an imprint of Perseus Books, LLC, a subsidiary of Hachette Book Group, Inc. The Running Press name and logo is a trademark of the Hachette Book Group.

The Hachette Speakers Bureau provides a wide range of authors for speaking events. To find out more, go to www.hachettespeakersbureau.com or call (866) 376-6591.

The publisher is not responsible for websites (or their content) that are not owned by the publisher.

Print book cover and interior by Josh McDonnell.

Library of Congress Control Number: 2018962790

ISBNs: 978-0-7624-6674-0 (paperback), 978-0-7624-6672-6 (ebook)

LSC-C

10 9 8 7 6 5 4 3 2 1

CONTENTS

INTRODUCTION

No, this book is not fiction. Running doesn't have to suck. But first things first. How do you currently feel about running?

- ☐ It sucks.
- ☐ I hate it.
- ☐ It hurts.
- ☐ It's boring.
- ☐ I'm afraid of it.
- ☐ I wish I could do it.
- ☐ I do it, but I hate it.
- ☐ I want to love it.
- ☐ All of the above. (Duh.)

Rest assured, you will feel differently about the negative answers—and closer to achieving the wishes and wants—even by the time you get to page 1 of this book. And you'll feel better still by the time you get to the end. Promise.

No matter what you answered above, *Running That Doesn't Suck* is for you. It's also for your friend, family member, coworker, neighbor, CrossFit buddy, yoga classmate, parent or teacher at your kids' school, or anyone you know who says they wish they liked running, but they hate it. (Go ahead and buy this book for them, too, to change their life.)

Running is hard. It hurts, especially at first. And it can hurt the second, third, fourth, and tenth time you try it if it's brand new to you, or if you've been forcing yourself to do it in a way that isn't true to who you are (see quiz on page xii!). But, for real, less suckiness *can* be achieved. Set out on a run using the tips in this book, and soon your perception of running will change. And then, magic: your body will hit a new gear. Your breathing will actually sync with the movement of your feet and your arms, and your brain will be loving your body for giving it a taste of that runner's high you thought was a myth.

And your body will be loving your brain for making you go.

Why do I know this? Because I love running, but I used to hate it. In high school, my hatred of running turned me into a sneak. I was on the track-and-field team, but as mostly a high jumper, and those big foam pits you land on after jumping over the high jump bar? They work great as hideout bunkers for teenagers who don't want to jog the two-lap team warm-up.

I played volleyball and soccer and had no problem chasing after a ball. On the track team, I did some sprinting and hurdling races, with the sight of a finish line no more than a hundred or two hundred yards away. But running any sort of long distance? I thought it sucked.

The summer before college, I had to change my ways. I planned on trying to walk on to my college volleyball team, and the coach had told me we had to run a sub-seven-minute timed mile.

Having been a California kid who'd grown up loving the beach, I figured I'd head down to Twenty-Fifth Street in Del Mar with my running shoes. (Any excuse to go to the beach.) I thought, *I'm an athlete; I can do this.*

I made it, maybe, to Twenty-Third Street. Two blocks.

I stopped, exasperated, exhausted, and annoyed. I walked a little. Then I looked down the beach and thought, *Make it to the next lifeguard tower,* which was another three blocks away. I don't think I made it that day without walking. But I kept going back, always eager to get to the place I loved, apprehensive about how far I'd get without having to walk.

On one of those early runs, I figured out to run down on the hard-packed sand, where the water laps the shore and creates a much harder—springy, even—surface than the deep stuff. And on one of those runs, I made it to that next lifeguard tower at Twentieth Street, then Seventeenth Street (eight whole blocks from where I started!). And I had a new goal: to make it to the next lifeguard tower, which was about two miles away on the next beach south.

That summer, I learned to love running. I started pushing my pace, trying to beat the setting sun. *Make it to that pile of seaweed before the sun dips fully into the horizon.* I got faster; I craved the motion of running. I made it to the tower on the next beach over and back, regularly. I went off to college, ran that sub-seven-minute mile, and walked on to the volleyball team. In fact, I ran the mile a lot better than I fared playing volleyball, and when I walked *off* the team that spring, I kept running.

Decades and thousands of miles later, I've spent years as a contributing editor to *Runner's World* and have been a running and outdoor sports journalist for twenty years. I've interviewed elite runners, amateur runners, running coaches, physiologists, sports psychologists, gait analysis experts, scientists studying effects of running, running specialty store owners and employees, running gear designers, and extraordinary folks of all sorts spanning the wide world of running. Over the course of my career, I've researched and written about everything from how to improve your speed, form, and joy while running to what to wear in virtually every degree of temperature, to the proper etiquette in nearly any running scenario you might find yourself in. I've written a trail running book called *Trailhead: The Dirt on All Things Trail Running.* I've run and raced and adventured around the world, and the blissfully simple movement of running is part of my identity. It's part of my soul. But I didn't always love it, and I'm on a mission to help others find the joy in it that I have.

I want to help you decode running, to stop being afraid of it, to stop hating it. It really doesn't have to suck. In fact, running can be awesome—you can love it!—if you approach it the right way.

This book is your key to unlocking that approach.

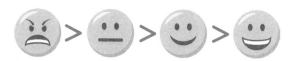

EMBRACE THE SUCKINESS

You may currently hate all runners, their short shorts and sports bras or nerdy singlets making you cringe. Runners tend to say things like "Running changed my life!" and "I feel so much better after I run!"—to which you may want to retort with things your mother probably wouldn't approve of.

That's okay. And also, don't worry—you don't have to wear split shorts and singlets (although you can if you want to). You'll see in Chapter 4 that running gear comes in all shapes and forms, from hipster cool to yoga-turned-running to full-on running geek. And you can talk about running however you want.

You probably also get tired of answering the question "Do you run?" with your go-to "Only if I'm being chased" line. Or you say something like "Running doesn't agree with this body," while you present your body with dramatic hand motions.

Maybe you have a bad association with running. Your junior high PE coach made you run laps for talking too much in class, or maybe you've tried to shed pounds by forcing yourself to run and it either didn't work or left a bad taste in your mouth (though perhaps that was the fat-free muffin you were making yourself eat). Maybe you think you will forever equate running with something negative.

But like any psychologist will tell you, it's healthy to embrace your emotions. It's okay to say you hate running, to admit that you think it sucks. But in doing so, know that you're one step away from changing how you feel about running. You're closer to moving past the "hate" emotion. And you *will* move past it with the pages of this book.

Read on. Your attitude toward running is about to change.

THE "LEARNING TO LOVE" PART

Think about the things in your life you look forward to doing. (Picture anything, even the perverted stuff. No one can see inside your brain.) Now think about how awesome it would be if running could become something you looked forward to doing. An activity you crave in mind, body, and spirit. Then it no longer becomes, *Ugh, I have to go work out*, but rather, *What time can I blow out of work so I can go run?* You no longer have to self-motivate. Your newfound love of running is motivating enough.

A 2016 study published in *Frontiers in Psychology* found that positive emotional reactions to certain types of exercise have a direct correlation to people sticking to that exercise long term.

This may sound obvious: Find a form of exercise you enjoy, and you'll stick with it. But so many people choose something they think they *have* to do to get fit, and they end up quitting because it just wasn't fun.

If you've picked up this book and have chosen running as your new form of exercise, or want to change your attitude about running for any reason at all, something inside you wants to love it. Keep reading, and this book will teach you *how* to love it.

WHAT DOES IT TAKE?

You may be reluctant to call anything you do, or have done in the past, "running." That's nonsense. Own it. Positive self-talk can do wonders. Here's what makes you a "runner" who can call what you do in a forward motion "running."

» **RUNNING.** That's what will make you a runner. Whether it's a half mile, a bunch of sprints on a football field, or five miles as fast as you can or as slow as anyone can imagine, you put one foot in front of the other in a pace faster than a walk, and you're a runner.

» **SHUFFLING.** If you don't consider your current form of running anything more than shuffling, you are now permitted to refer to your shuffling as running.

» **RUN/WALKING.** Heading out and walking for a good chunk of your "run"—even running for just thirty seconds at a time interspersed with walking breaks—makes you a runner. See page 115 for training plans that combine running and walking.

TRUST THE PROCESS

"When you're a new runner, it's hard to imagine that you'll one day love and be addicted to running. Likewise, if you're in a running slump, it seems impossible that you'll ever get back to enjoying running again. But you will! Each step you take forward adds up until you love running and need to have it in your life. Just keep at it; the love and addiction will build."

—Kara Goucher, two-time Olympian and author of *Strong: A Runner's Guide to Boosting Confidence and Becoming the Best Version of You*

SMELLING THE FLOWERS WITH MIRNA VALERIO

Mirna Valerio, accomplished ultramarathoner and author of the blog *Fat Girl Running* and the book *Beautiful Work in Progress*, advocates that everyone can run. "You don't have to be super fast; you can run at your own pace," she says. "You can stop and smell the flowers and then start running again. There are so many different ways to exist in running."

She adds, "Once you start accepting where you are as a runner, then it becomes easier. It becomes more doable."

THE MASTER KEY: KNOW THYSELF

Knowing yourself well is the key to successfully navigating so many aspects of life. Know girls'/boys' nights out are overwhelming to you? Don't go, and catch up with your friends in small groups. Know you shouldn't lead a work meeting unless you drink a double espresso? Head to the coffee shop and start pounding.

If you've tried to become a runner in the past but got frustrated and quit somewhere in the process, chances are you were forcing yourself to run in ways—times of the day, locations or types of surfaces, in certain company—that didn't mesh well with your personality.

For instance, if you're the type of person who craves nature, forcing yourself to run on concrete or on a treadmill likely won't make you fall in love with running, but trail running would. And if you're a gym rat or ex–field sport athlete who loves going fast for short amounts of time, running track intervals with a running club might be the perfect scenario for you.

Knowing yourself—and acting on that knowledge—transcends all when it comes to making running not suck. To home in on what might work best for you in your pursuit of learning to love running, take the "Know-Thyself-to-Become-a-Runner" quiz on page xii.

The rest of the book will unlock wisdom and advice to help you set your unique self up for successful, non-sucky running.

HOW TO USE THIS BOOK

After the ever-so-valuable "Know-Thyself-to-Become-a-Runner" quiz on page xii, this book is broken down into ten chapters that you do not need to read in order. Your answers to the quiz will direct you to certain chapters for more information on specific topics, and the rest of the book serves up further information and advice that can help anyone love running more. Seriously.

Feel free to flip to a specific chapter—like when you're looking for a no-nonsense guide on what running shoes to buy (page 59) or a good stretch to coax a certain ache to go away (page 144), or read this cover to cover for an overall shift in how you approach—and more important, perceive—running. (Plus, inspiration and jokes.)

In the pages to come, you'll discover why, with what, with whom, where, and specifically *how* running can work for you. You'll learn how to take care of your body so you don't break down (and so you can't use that as an excuse to quit). You'll discover why your knees (and other body parts) might hurt and how to make them stop hurting. You'll learn about nutrition, etiquette, and setting flexible goals.

But this is not your standard beginner's running book. It is not normal. Because we are acknowledging off the bat, here and now, that you currently hate the feeling—and maybe even the thought of—moving your feet one in front of the other, slightly off the ground one at a time.

In fact, the following chapters are broken down by reasons you might have for hating running, then go on to turn those negative feelings on their heads. We'll zap each one until you're out of ~~excuses~~ reasons.

Yes, the following pages will help you find that love of running. You no longer have to dread it, or hate it, or swear every time the word *running* comes up. You can love it. It doesn't have to suck.

THE KNOW-THYSELF-TO-BECOME-A-RUNNER QUIZ

A little self-knowledge can go a long way and can help set you up for success. This quiz will help start you on your path to becoming someone who loves running. For real.

1. Are you a morning person?

YES. Consider running first thing in the morning.

NO. Don't force yourself to run first thing in the morning, or you're bound to hate it. Schedule your run for later in the day.

For more on how to successfully get out the door any time of day, see Chapter 2.

2. If you don't work out first thing in the morning, will you freak out all day that you haven't gone?

YES. Run in the morning so you're more pleasant to be around all day.

NO. Run whenever you can, and revel in your easygoing nature.

For more on managing your time (and digestive system) to run at any time of day, see Chapter 2.

3. Do you suffer from high stress or are prone to anxiety?

YES. Consider running later in the day to help blow off steam, mitigate anxiety, and help you fall asleep by clearing your mind.

NO. Run whenever, you lucky bastard.

For yet even more on running all times of the day, see Chapter 2.

4. Are you an introvert?

YES. Run with others sometimes, but set aside some runs for just you and your thoughts. You'll learn to cherish—and crave—that kind of alone time . . . in motion.

NO. Pair up with a running buddy or running group for social motivation. And if you loved playing team sports as a kid, consider joining a running club.

For more on the pros and cons of running with partners, clubs, groups, or dogs, or running solo, see Chapter 5.

5. **Are you an animal lover or natural-born caregiver?**

YES. Consider running with a dog. The caregiver in you will be motivated by your dog's need for exercise.

NO. You selfish jerk. Just kidding. Try not to spit on the squirrels you pass by when you run by yourself.

For more on running with a dog, see Chapter 5.

6. **Are you a nature lover?**

YES. If you love being outside—hiking, gardening, bird-watching, mountain biking, or doing other activities related to dirt—try trail running (especially if road or treadmill running doesn't do it for you).

NO. If you're more inspired by the thought of logging meditative—or just plain fast—miles on the roads, or if you want to ease into running in the comfort of your gym, kick off your running there.

For more on where to run to never be bored, see Chapters 2 and 3.

7. **Are you supercompetitive?**

YES. You'll likely be inspired by socially competitive apps or races. Just wait until you're a few months in to start comparing yourself to others, or you might get pissed off and lose motivation. Also, envision yourself racing once you get used to running. Your competitive self will eat that shit up.

NO. Stay away from stopwatches and said apps, and consider jumping into races for fun and motivation, even when you're just starting out. (But don't think you need to race to be a runner. You don't.) Seek out training apps that log your progress and map your runs instead of apps that compare your runs to other people's.

For more on training/competitive apps, see Chapter 4. For more on racing, see Chapter 10.

8. Are you driven by technology?

YES. You're in luck. There is an insane number of techy wrist computers that track everything from pace, to foot strike, to distance, to how well you sleep. You'll find motivation in getting one of these things and geeking out.

NO. For you, simplicity rules. Consider going running without even a wrist-watch, and listen to your body. Go by feel. You don't need to tech-out to be a runner.

For more on options for what to wear on your wrist, see Chapter 4.

9. Are you a music lover or podcast fan, or can you never find enough time to listen to audiobooks?

YES. One word: headphones! Throw on a pair of headphones, and hit the road. Pump music that fires you up, learn something fascinating during a podcast, or "read" a book while you run.

NO. You may also have answered yes to number 6, in which case you'll likely prefer the sounds of birds chirping, wind rustling, and leaves crunching beneath your feet, and the rhythm of your own breath. Leave the headphones at home and consider running in nature for inspiring, meditative ambient sound.

See Chapters 4 and 5 for more on headphones (and safety precautions for running while wearing them), and music player/phone-carrying devices.

10. Are you intimidated by where to run?

YES. That's totally okay. If the thought of exploring your neighborhood or a trail solo and by foot freaks you out, run with a friend or a club. If you'd prefer the predictable, hit a track or treadmill.

NO. Embrace your inner explorer. Running new routes—whether they're in a city you're visiting or in your own neighborhood can open up a world of possible running routes and be extremely motivating.

Turn to page 84 for how to find a running club and page 88 for how find a running partner. For track and treadmill survival guides see pages 26 and 28, and check out Chapters 2 and 5 for how to safely explore while you run.

You get an A+ for answering the above questions honestly and getting one step closer to actually enjoying running. Maybe some of these options even got you excited to try a different approach to becoming the runner you want to be. Get ready to really discover what will work best for you to make running not suck, once and for all.

TEN KEYS TO NON-SUCKY RUNNING

With knowing thyself being the master key that unlocks a new world of non-suckiness, the following chapters will give you ten actionable keys to unlock individual doors to success. Whenever you see this, know that there is a pearl of wisdom wrapped up into four words or less that will help you start loving running. Really. The ten keys will be discussed in the chapters ahead.

"Why bother?"

FIND YOUR REASON TO RUN

*S*ure, there are a million body benefits to running, *blah, blah, blah,* that we'll get to later. But what if your main reason for becoming a runner was how it makes you *feel* instead of how it makes you look?

Wouldn't that just turn your perspective on running on its head?

How awesome would it be to approach running like a kid—to want to run because it's fun? Or to actually *crave* running because the steady, rhythmic motion makes you feel good? Even a short run can change your mood for the better, reset your day, and help you make big decisions purely because you're in motion and your brain works differently on a run than when you're sitting at your desk. Focus on how running can make you feel, and the body benefits will come. That mind shift alone will make running way more appealing—and maybe even a little easier.

VISUALIZATION AS MOTIVATION

"Visualization is a powerful tool," says Dr. Stephen Walker, sports psychologist and athletic and performance consultant.

Walker explains there are three pieces to utilizing visualization to help get you out the door. "One is to visualize your goal in terms of it being easy for you to get out there and enjoy the run in the way that you want to, once the momentum kicks in and you feel good," he says. "Then visualize how good it feels after your run, having accomplished what you did and appreciating and enjoying how relaxed you are after working out the kinks on your run." And thirdly, "Visualize how your clothes will fit differently as you stick with running. How you feel stronger, more capable, and more powerful while doing everything you need to do in your life."

GET ALL MIND-BODY ON IT

The notion of the mind-body connection in today's psychology circles means that the mind and body are linked and can affect each other—for the worse, like in the case of stress-induced illnesses, but also for the better, like how improved posture can boost confidence. And since running can give you greater feelings of self-worth, an enhanced mood, and more energy, there's an inverse relationship at play, too. These benefits make up the elusive, oft-touted runner's high that's a big part of getting—and keeping—you hooked.

DRUG HIGH VERSUS THE RUNNER'S HIGH

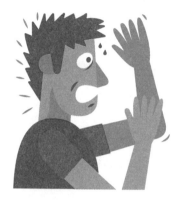 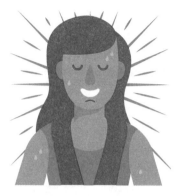

DRUG HIGH

ELATION: Short term

HAZARDS: Bad for your health. Spend all your money on drugs. Hangover is terrible.

RUNNER'S HIGH

ELATION: Long term.

HAZARDS: Zilch.

RUNNER'S HIGH: WHAT THE HELL IS IT, AND HOW DO YOU GET IT?

Maybe you've heard about the runner's high, but as far as you're concerned, it's an elusive load of hoo-ha a running gear company made up to get you to buy stuff.

The runner's high is the crack runners seek. The feeling runners crave. The high that gets some runners out the door at 5:00 a.m., day after day, or that motivates a runner to change clothes at lunchtime to return to work with dried sweat in his hair. It's the euphoria that sends a mom of four to the garage for a treadmill run after her kids are in bed.

WHAT SCIENCE SAYS ABOUT THE RUNNER'S HIGH

The runner's high is also very real. Its power can be attributed to these elements:

ENDORPHINS!

It's well known at this point that when you exercise, your body releases chemicals called *endorphins*. And studies suggest that the more endorphins released into the brain due to running, the better subjects felt.

What are endorphins? The very word is made up of the root words *endogenous* (coming from within an organism) and *morphine* (a pain medication). Basically, they're natural painkillers your body makes itself. Pretty cool.

ENDOCANNABIS!

A 2015 study published in the *Proceedings of the National Academy of Sciences* likened the blissed-out runner's high to the high marijuana smokers experience. The study demonstrated that cannabinoid receptors, which help regulate pain and anxiety, are heightened by running. Cue up jokes about giggling, mellow potheads.

OPIOIDS!

A 2008 study published in *Cerebral Cortex* found that the "level of euphoria was significantly increased after running" and that the findings support the "'opioid theory' of the runner's high and suggest region-specific effects in frontolimbic brain areas that are involved in the processing of affective states and mood." Opioids are generally used in medicine as pain relievers. This study suggests that our bodies produce our own when running.

ANTIDEPRESSANT!

A 2007 study in the *American College of Sports Medicine's Health & Fitness Journal* even found that an exercise program "was just as effective as prescription anti-depressants in patients with major depressive disorder." And while this one studied exercise programs in the general sense, running was part of that program.

That's all to say that the runner's high makes you feel damn good. Things that feel good become addictive.

Get addicted to the feeling, and you'll want to keep doing it, like that lady at work who stands at the watercooler and says things like "My husband knows I need to get my run in or else I'm a real B." (Maybe soon *you'll* need a run "or else . . ."!)

A POSITIVE ADDICTION

The book *Positive Addiction* by psychiatrist Dr. William Glasser states that said good addictions "strengthen us and make our lives more satisfying." They also enable us to "live with more confidence, more creativity, and more happiness, and usually in much better health."

Doesn't that sound f***ing great? What if your positive addiction to running gave you all that?

HOW SOON CAN I GET IT?

How far—or how fast—do you have to run to get the drug-like runner's high? Not very.

"Most of the data suggests that you need to be running for at least thirty minutes or more before a runner's high can kick in," says Steve Magness, coach, exercise physiologist, and author of *Peak Performance: Elevate Your Game, Avoid Burnout, and Thrive with the New Science of Success.* "We need to go just hard enough where we have to be engaged and our attention is in the moment, but not so hard that fatigue and effort are overwhelming us." He adds, "There's a lot of variation because what is comfortably challenging for one will be short and easy for another. What we are clear on is that it won't happen a few minutes into a jog down the street."

The takeaway? Work toward a thirty-minute run, stick with it, and be patient. The runner's high will come.

MINDFUL OR MINDLESS RUNNING?

Some believe that the fastest way to achieve the runner's high is to be mindful while running. Others are motivated by distractions—music, thoughts, whatever. Here's a look at the merits of mindful and mindless running, and how to achieve either.

MINDFUL RUNNING

"Runners tend to feel the best after runs during which they spent time in the flow state, also known as getting 'in the zone,'" says Mackenzie Havey, author of *Mindful Running: How Meditative Running Can Improve Performance and Make You a Happier, More Fulfilled Person*. "By being totally focused on the present moment, unproductive and distracting thoughts are limited and you run and feel your best. It is after these runs that runners often experience the runner's high."

HOW TO DO IT: Focus on your five senses. See your surroundings. Listen to your breath, the wind, the birds. Smell the fresh air and trees. Feel your body. Taste . . . well, be aware of the taste in your mouth. Do this for a few minutes each run, working up to longer periods of meditative running.

THE POINT is to be present. Focus on the moment, and clear your mind.

MINDLESS RUNNING

"I need my f***ing headphones blasting music or else I won't make it half a mile on a run," says the proponent of mindless running.

HOW TO DO IT: Let your mind wander and think all the crazy thoughts you want—or wear headphones and zone out listening to distracting music or a podcast. Loophole: Havey says that listening to repetitive, zone-out music (like music without lyrics, or music you know by heart) can allow for mindful running, so if you're aiming for mindlessness, avoid techno or the *Frozen* soundtrack (yeah, you, parents of little girls).

THE POINT is to get out the door, and if being totally distracted with music or anything filling your ears through headphones—or working through thoughts without headphones—is what gets you to do that, then embrace the mindlessness (but consider dabbling in mindfulness to see how it makes you feel).

THE GRAVY: BODY BENEFITS

Warning: While reading this section, do not lose sight of the main motivating factor to start running, which is how it makes you feel (not look). The body benefits are the gravy. The icing on the cake. The gravy on the icing on the cake.

That said, get ready to look awesome. Visualizing this awesomeness—the future you—does have powerful, motivating effects not to be discounted.

PUBLIC SERVICE ANNOUNCEMENT

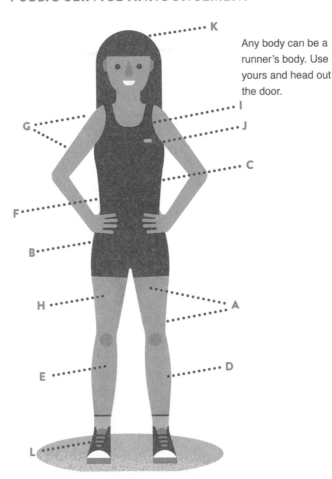

Any body can be a runner's body. Use yours and head out the door.

PARTS OF YOU THAT WILL BE STRONGER

A. THIGHS/QUADS

» With every single running step, you strengthen your quadriceps muscles, which are those sexy, strong muscles on the front of your thighs. Strengthening these long muscles, combined with torching calories, helps your thighs move farther apart from each other.

» **Benefits of strong quads:** Kicking soccer balls. Climbing stairs. Feeling stronger with every step.

B. BUTT

» Running engages all the butt muscles—the gluteus medius, maximus, and minimus—and firms that backside right up.

» **Benefits of a strong butt:** Keeping your jeans from falling down. Dominating musical chairs. Supporting your abs and core.

C. AB MUSCLES

» Running, by way of burning calories (see sidebar), helps shrink your waistline and define your abdominal wall. Trail running, especially, requires balance to stay upright as you negotiate rocks and other terrain obstacles, meaning your core gets stronger with every step. Exercises like planks can help strengthen your core, which will in turn help you become a better runner (and be more spring break ready).

» **Benefits of having strong abs:** Preventing injuries in day-to-day life. Standing more upright. Looking gooood.

D. SHINS

» You know that muscle that shows up (or is supposed to show up, or used to show up) on your shin when you flex your toes? That muscle—the tibialis anterior—becomes defined on runners. It's kind of rad.

» **Benefits of a strong tibialis:** Not falling off balance beams. Feeling more agile. Having better coordination.

E. CALVES

» Running uphill, in particular, defines calves—the gastrocnemius muscles—unlike anything else (aside from thousands of box jumps or calf raises).

» **Benefits of strong calves:** Minimizing ankle, foot, and knee injuries. Reaching something on the top shelf of your kitchen with ease. Running and walking with more power, especially uphill.

CALORIE BURNER

How many calories does running burn? There's an old estimate that says we burn roughly one hundred calories per mile, but certain factors change this number. For instance:

- The more you weigh, the more you burn.
- The faster you run, the more you burn.
- The higher your individual metabolism, the more you burn.

Wherever you fall among the above factors, know that running is one of the best calorie torchers out there. See Chapter 8 for more information.

PARTS OF YOU THAT WILL LOOK SMALLER

F. WAISTLINE

» Yes, your waistline will shrink. Inches will fall off you as you ramp up your running. See "Calorie Burner" sidebar.

G. SHOULDERS/ARMS

» Truth be told, running doesn't do a lot for the upper body, aside from slim it down from the overall calorie torching.

Sure, your butt, legs, and so on will likely look smaller, too, but the important thing here is that they will be stronger and enable you to feel more like an indestructible superhero.

MYSTERIOUS WEIGHT GAIN

Some people experience weight gain, instead of loss, when starting to run . . . which can really piss a person off. Sometimes, that gain is due to changes in body composition; we've all heard that muscle weighs more than fat, and as you run more and get stronger, you'll be losing fat and gaining muscle. But some new runners' weight gain can be attributed to an increase in appetite due to all that calorie burning and eating way more because of it. Which is okay! Once you start including added challenges like hills and different paces to your runs and focusing on foods that repair muscles post-run, that new weight usually falls right off. (See Chapter 8 for pointers on nutrition.)

PARTS YOU CAN'T SEE (BUT YOU CAN FEEL)

H. BONES

» Low-impact exercises like swimming and biking are great for you, but the impact of running has a big upside because it can strengthen your bones, even helping to ward off osteoporosis and preserve bone marrow. A 2009 study in the *Journal of Strength and Conditioning Research* concluded, "Both resistance training and high-impact endurance activities increase bone mineral density. However, high-impact sports, like running, appear to have a greater beneficial effect." And a 2018 Australian study published in the *Journal of Bone and Mineral Research* found that running actually preserves bone marrow. Think of running as weight training for your bones—just as lifting dumbbells helps encourage muscle growth, the impact of each step while running helps prompt bones to increase their density.

» **Benefit of strong bones:** Not breaking them. Less shrinking with age.

I. HEART

» Running improves blood flow. It also lowers your resting heart rate, which makes your heart's job easier. That's why doctors often recommend physical exercise for heart health. A 2017 study published in the medical journal *Progress in Cardiovascular Diseases* even claimed that runners live three years longer than non-runners. (Your results may vary.)

» **Benefit of having a healthy heart:** Not dying too soon.

J. LUNGS

» In 2016, the Lung Institute put out an article citing the benefits of exercise, stating that "lung capacity can be controlled and improved 5 to 15% through aerobic exercise." The article explains that while training your aerobic system (with cardiovascular exercise like—you guessed it—running) can't improve lung function (how much air your body can hold), "training can improve endurance and reduce breathlessness by increasing oxygen capacity."

» **Benefit of improved lung capacity:** Less breathlessness while chasing kids around, running to the bus stop, and doing virtually anything.

K. BRAIN

» As mentioned earlier in this chapter, running creates all sorts of positive chemical reactions in the brain. It's a downright natural high.

» **Benefit of a healthy brain:** What *isn't* a benefit of a healthy brain?

L. FEET

» Feet can't really be seen when you're running, unless, of course, you're running barefoot . . . which, incidentally, strengthens feet.[1] The benefits of strong foot muscles and bones don't stop at the ankle; strong feet send support upward through your lower legs, knees, upper legs, hips, back, and so on. If you discover that you need or prefer running shoes with cushioning and/or support (see Chapter 4), strengthen feet by walking around your house and outside barefoot, and/or do the exercises on page 139 for strong tootsies.

» **Benefits of having strong feet:** Injury prevention. Winning money off bets that you can't write your name with your toes.

---

1   This statement is fully loaded. If you're curious about barefoot running, pick up a book dedicated to the subject and ease into the method one step at a time. Like, literally, one step at a time—it takes some serious getting used to and is not recommended without a very cautious plan and guidance.

RUNNING AND KNEES

Running gets a bad rap when it comes to knees. But a 2008 study done at Stanford University debunked the myth that running causes osteoarthritic knees and actually supported that cartilage can be trained in positive patterns by walking and running. A 2008 paper published In *Skeletal Radiology* stated that no knee damage was found in six of seven runners who had raced in marathons for ten years. And a 2017 study published in the *European Journal of Applied Physiology* pointed to running decreasing inflammation in the knee. For more on keeping knees healthy while running, see pages 143 to 147.

KEY NO. 1 TO MAKING RUNNING NOT SUCK: VISUALIZE THE NEW YOU

Use the power of your brain to imagine how awesome you'll feel after a run and, ahem, look after a few weeks of running. Use that image in your brain to get you out the door . . . and then get out the door. You'll soon become addicted to the feeling. Keep visualizing it.

Sucky thought zapped by this chapter:

"I have no reason to start running."

"No time. No place to go."

FIGURE OUT WHEN AND WHERE

How on earth do you get started, or how on earth do you restart a running routine that you currently hate? Whether running is brand new to you, or you're attempting a rebirth, knowing the where and when that works best for you—and specifically you—can make a world of difference.

Let's figure out where and when you can go to transform yourself into someone who loves running.

KEY NO. 2 TO MAKING RUNNING NOT SUCK: FIND YOUR FLOW

Since there are no two humans alike, there is no single time of day or singular location for a run that is ideal for everyone. Homing in on your personal preferences for time and place will help you find your flow as a runner and set you up for successfully continuing to be a runner.

FIGURING OUT WHEN TO RUN

There is no magic hour that works for all runners. Yes, there are those chipper folks who have run and showered by 7:00 a.m. and have the whole day ahead of them. But finding the perfect time of day to run is an individual matter.

In the quiz on pages xii through xiv, you answered a few questions about what times of day might work for you as a runner, based on various factors. How you answered those questions—and will answer a few more in the flowchart that follows—will help you zero in on what time of day to try to kick off your successful transition to becoming a runner.

MORNING RUN?
SET YOURSELF UP FOR SUCCESS

There's more to becoming a morning runner than just . . . running in the morning. There's the whole *how to make it happen* thing. If you're going in the morning, you'll want to experiment with how much time you need before a run. Do you need to get up an hour ahead of time to eat breakfast, have coffee, and poop? Or can you wake up and run and do all that stuff when you get home?

Let's troubleshoot some common problems you might come across with morning runs.

1. **The issue:** You have to stop for a poop break mid-run.

   » **Solution:** Get up earlier, have coffee or tea, let your body have time to do its thing.

2. **The issue:** You're pissed off that you're up early eating breakfast, prepping for what seems like forever, for a run.

» **Solution:** Set your alarm for just a few minutes before you plan on running. Consider sleeping in your running socks and even in your running clothes. (Women: Know that sleeping in running shorts ups a risk for a yeast infection. Also know that sleeping in a sports bra can hinder certain evening pastimes, so use that knowledge as you will.) Place your running shoes by the door. Get up, skip breakfast and coffee or tea, and head out the door ASAP. (If issue No. 1 arises, find a middle ground.)

TO-DO LIST THE NIGHT BEFORE A MORNING RUN:

☐ Eat a big dinner and drink plenty of water (or a water chaser after you're done with your cocktail).

☐ Check the weather forecast for the hour you'll be running in the morning, then select running outfit: bottom, top, sports bra (if applicable), socks, shoes. Accessories: sunglasses, hat, gloves, phone-carrying device, headlamp (if applicable). Winter running add-ons: gloves, beanie, jacket. For more on what to wear in what scenarios, see Chapter 4.

☐ Put said items out in a room where no one sleeps so you don't disturb your bedmate, even if that bedmate is a cat.

☐ Set your alarm *without* the snooze option.

☐ Go to sleep. If you have a hard time sleeping because of your looming morning run, consider the three Ms: melatonin, meditating, or making yourself a cup of tea.

TO-DO LIST THE MORNING OF A RUN:

☐ Get up. Go. Refer back to potential issues No. 1 and 2.

> **Motivational tip:** Think of the runner's high you're trying to get addicted to. Think of the hot shower you'll have when you get home. Visualize your new self. Visualize how great of a day you'll have following your morning run.

MIDDAY RUNNER?
SET YOURSELF UP FOR SUCCESS

It's true: not everyone can pull off a run midday. But if you work in an environment that A) has a shower; B) Is casual (enough); C) is with coworkers who don't mind sweat drying in your hair; all combined with D) the ability to head out the door for thirty minutes to an hour for a midday break, then running midday could be a time-saver for you. It can also be a good way to rejuvenate your afternoon. Instead of dragging and pounding caffeine after lunch, you'll be buzzing naturally from your run. Plus, running with a coworker or two or more can be great bonding. (And you can gossip about your other coworkers while running.)

Let's troubleshoot some common problems you might come across with midday runs.

1. **The issue:** You don't know where to go.

   » **Solution:** Ask among officemates to see if anyone runs, and if so, where. Or get an officemate to go exploring with you. Or use one of a number of apps available to find popular running routes near your office.

2. **The issue:** You like lunch.

   » **Solution:** Pack a lunch at home and eat it at your desk after your run. If you're starving on your actual run-lunch (which you can jokingly call *runch* for now on), have an easy-to-digest snack like a banana or other simple carbs at your desk at least an hour before your run.

3. **The issue:** You sweat.

   » **Solution:** Either your office has a shower you can use and change back into your work clothes, or you're screwed. (Kidding.) If you don't have access to a shower, consider wiping down with baby wipes, sport wipes made specifically for this purpose, or a good, old-fashioned washcloth and soap and water, and reapply deodorant or antiperspirant. Even if you don't have a shower and do the wipe-down method, consider bringing a hair dryer to dry sweat. (Your hair will be fine. It's good to not over-wash it anyway, and dried sweat can actually work like natural hair product.)

» Or, if you have access to a nearby gym, you could either run outside or inside on the gym's treadmill and take a shower there before returning to work.

TO-DO LIST THE MORNING OF A MIDDAY RUN:
- ☐ Eat a substantial breakfast, and consider having a snack midmorning.
- ☐ Pack lunch and bring it to work.
- ☐ Pack running clothes and shoes (after checking weather).
- ☐ If you have an office shower, pack towel and toiletries (and rubber flip-flops for the shower—otherwise, yuck).
- ☐ If no shower, pack baby or sport wipes or a washcloth, maybe a hair dryer.

> **Motivational tip:** Know how good you'll feel after your run, and after work, knowing you already got your exercise. (Woohoo, happy hour!) Also, your coworkers will start noticing your midday runs and may join you . . . or just appreciate your calm afternoon demeanor while thinking you're a badass.

END-OF-DAY RUN?
SET YOURSELF UP FOR SUCCESS

Running at the end of the day can be hard for some people. Finding the energy after a day of work or school or—toughest of all—being a parent to young kids can seem impossible. But running at the end of the day and shaking the day's stresses can provide a welcome change of gears and send you coasting into a relaxing evening.

You got it—it's troubleshooting time.

1. **The issue:** You're tired.

   » **Solution:** Know that there's nothing like a few minutes into a run (or run/walk) to wake you up. Unless you're in the middle of a multiday run across, say, the Gobi Desert, it is nearly impossible to fall asleep while running. If you're really dragging in the afternoon, consider caffeine at least an hour before you plan to go.

2. **The issue:** You're a responsible adult.

   » **Solution:** You may have dinner to cook, errands to run, and/or children to cart around to various sporting events, but there are ways to squeeze in the end-of-day run: if your work is semi-close to home, consider the run/walk commute; if you're stuck at a ball field or sports venue of some sort after driving the carpool, do some laps around the fields; if you can run on your way home from work (before you get home and your sweats and glass of wine tempt you), do that; if you have a friend who can commit to running with you, or meet a running group after work (see page 84), do it (especially if your run is after dark).

TO-DO LIST LEADING UP TO AN END-OF-DAY RUN:

- ☐ Eat a substantial breakfast.
- ☐ Pack your running clothes and bring them to work.
- ☐ Eat a substantial lunch.
- ☐ Eat a late-afternoon snack, something that's easy to digest—think plain bagel, not a plate of nachos.
- ☐ Consider late-afternoon caffeine, but not if it keeps you up all night.
- ☐ Look forward to your run all day.
- ☐ If you're running at the end of the day and it'll be dark, be sure to wear a headlamp, handheld light, or reflective clothing (see page 80).

> **Motivational tip:** Visualize shaking the day's stresses and easing into your evening in a more blissed-out state.

THE WHEN-TO-RUN FLOWCHART

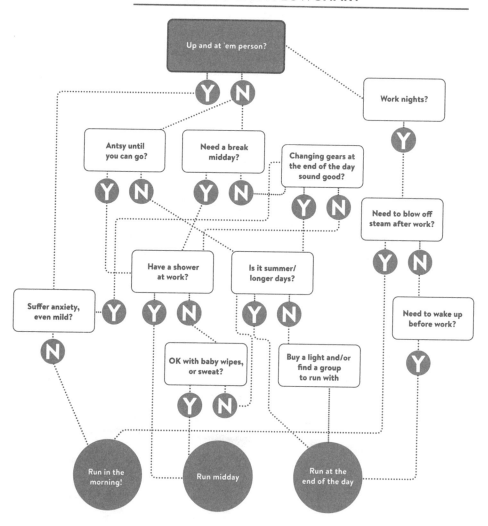

Now that you've followed the path to find your own answer, don't put off your first run/walk until next Tuesday. Do it in the next open window. Do it. (See page 24 for where to do it and Chapter 6 to see for how long you should do it.)

FIGURING OUT WHERE TO RUN

Just as running at certain times of the day is an individual matter, finding a running environment that works specifically for you can make a huge difference in whether you can learn to love running or will forever think it sucks.

The quiz on page xii had you answer a few questions about personal preferences—natural environments or controlled situations, for instance. How you answered those questions—and will answer a few more in the flowchart that follows—will help you figure out where running will be most enjoyable for *you*.

THE WHERE-TO-RUN FLOWCHART

Everybody's different, and you may feel differently day-to-day and can try all scenarios. In fact, mixing things up is encouraged. (More on this on page 25.) But to figure out in what type of environment to kick off your successful life as a runner, start with where you ended up by following the above, and then check out the Choose Your Own Adventure–style Chapter 3 to learn more about what to expect in each type of environment.

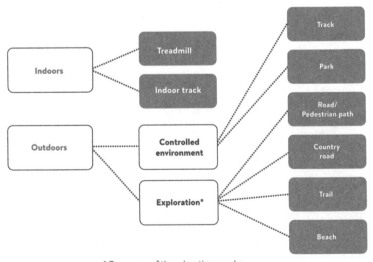

* Even some of these locations can be controlled by running out and back.

TRAILS/URBAN TRAILS: WHY/HOW/WHERE

Trail does not have to mean a harrowing single-track path where you're dangling off a cliff. Nor does it mean a big-mountain adventure with summits, snowstorms, and grizzlies. A trail can be a flat, wide, dirt path and still deliver the benefits of trail running.

WHY TRAILS?

Studies have proven the mind-body benefits of exercising in nature, and you don't get more nature-y than a trail. Running on a trail builds core strength with all those little (and big) muscles working to keep you stable. And running on a trail is fun—it can release your inner adventurer/inner child.

HOW TO FIND A TRAIL/URBAN TRAIL

- **Ask a friend!** Be sure to let your friend know you're looking for a smooth, mellow trail for starters (if you are).
- **Ask a running or outdoor shop employee!** Be sure to let this person know you're looking for a smooth, mellow trail for starters (if you are).
- **Join a running club!** Running clubs often meet at various trails, giving you a safe environment to explore trails in a group and return to them solo. (See page 84 for more on running clubs.)
- **Search online!** The internet is amazing. Type *running/hiking/mountain biking trails in whereveryoulive*, and a plethora of information will magically appear.
- **Go exploring!** Cruising around your neighborhood looking for dirt, wood chips, or grass can be fun, and it can lead you to a whole world of natural paths you didn't know existed.

HOW TO MAKE SURE YOU ENJOY IT

Go with someone who knows the trail. Bring a map (and know that digital maps on phones aren't fail-safe), or at least look at one before you head out. Do a simple, straightforward out-and-back run/walk the first few times you go. No turns! If you ignore this warning and make turns, pay close attention and even look behind you to memorize what that turn will look like on your way back.

See page 190 for more about trail running.

> **TIP: MIX IT UP**
>
> If you ever get bored with one location and running just becomes *sooo* boring, change it up. Get out of your neighborhood and go run in someone else's neighborhood. If you get tired of roads, try a smooth dirt trail. If a treadmill is making you feel like a hamster on a wheel, run outside, even around your gym.

CHASING BEAUTY

"When I was running for weight loss, I felt like I could never let myself walk. But once I started to switch over to running on trails—something that was fun and beautiful—I realized walking was not a failure. I realized that trail running doesn't have to mean you're running every second from start to finish. The trails here in Portland are so beautiful that runs are no longer a workout, necessarily. It's like, 'Let's go hike . . . but faster.' I think that started to switch my mind-set."

—Shane Upchurch, 35, Portland, Oregon

CITY PARKS/BALL FIELDS/TRACKS: WHY/HOW/WHERE

City parks, ball fields, and tracks can provide great natural settings and surfaces if you run on grass or dirt, without having to worry about getting lost (unless, of course, you're in a really big park).

WHY PARKS/FIELDS/TRACKS?

Most city parks, large or small, have either grass or paved pedestrian paths—both of which can be great for running. Ball fields can be great for the same reason, and for the added bonus of getting in a run while your kid practices his or her sport, or . . . running on an empty field just gives you a pleasant place to run. Tracks can: A) drive a person insane; B) be great for safe, brainless running— you're not gonna get lost; C) be the home of your first speed-work session. Fun! (See page 203.)

HOW TO FIND A PARK/FIELD/TRACK

» **Look at a map.** When looking at a map, either printed or online, look for green spaces. See them as green squares or rectangles of possibility for pleasant running. Reddish or blackish ovals on Google Maps or Google Earth are likely tracks.

» **Search the web.** Look for schools in your area, and dig deeper to find out if those schools have tracks. Dig even deeper to see if those tracks have open hours for non-students.

» **Keep your eyes peeled.** In your car, on your bike, or on your feet, keep an eye out for green spaces and tracks, and return with your running shoes.

HOW TO MAKE SURE YOU ENJOY IT

If you're running around a small park, a ball field, or a track, know that you'll be making turns to one side during your run. To avoid an overuse injury from making all left turns, for instance, change direction the next time you run there to help balance out your muscles on both sides of your body. See Chapter 3 for more on running in parks, around fields, and on tracks. And see Chapter 9 for track etiquette.

URBAN PATHS/NEIGHBORHOODS/ROADS: WHY/HOW/WHERE

Running straight from home is the most convenient way to get a run in, for most people. If you're lucky, your neighborhood has sidewalks. If not, take extra safety measures. And either way, seek out urban pedestrian paths for car- and bike-free running.

WHY A PATH/NEIGHBORHOOD/ROAD

Convenience rules. Also, urban pedestrian paths let you run without worrying about cars backing out of their driveways, running in traffic, or halting at stoplights.

HOW TO FIND A PATH/ROUTE

Run out your door and around the block (if you live on a block), increasing your range each time you head out.

Run out the door, and run in one direction for a set amount of time or to a certain landmark, then turn around and retrace your steps.

Do a web search for pedestrian-only paths in your area.

Explore potential running routes via car or, better yet, bike.

HOW TO MAKE SURE YOU ENJOY IT

If you find yourself running on a road without sidewalks, run facing traffic and as far to the side of the road as possible. If the road turns and you're running into a blind corner, cross the street when you're sure no cars are coming and run on the other side until it's safe to cross back over. Also, if you must run with headphones, keep one earbud out or the volume low; you want to be able to hear cars, bikes, other runners, and so on. Safety first. For more on paths and other paved routes, see Chapter 3.

> **TIP: GO EXPLORING**
> If you still find yourself getting bored, get your hands on some maps of your neighborhood and/or nearby open space. Maps are like portals to new running adventures. See page 40 about how to not get lost. And see Chapter 3 to forever beat boredom.

TREADMILLS: WHY/HOW/WHERE

Few people ever fell in love with running on a treadmill. But treadmills don't always deserve to be called "dreadmills."

WHY A TREADMILL?

Circumstances where a treadmill is the best place to run:

- You're intimidated by where to go. (Okay for now, but after a few treadmill runs, brave the great outdoors.)
- You're injured, or coming back from an injury, and don't know how long you can run. (It's a lot easier to step off a treadmill and end your run than it is to hobble home from a mile or two away if something flares up.)
- Your kids are in the gym day care. Some gyms don't let you leave the premises if your kids are in their day care, so a treadmill might be your only option for getting in a run.

- Your baby is asleep in a bucket car seat next to the treadmill. You'll be able to keep an eye on him or her. If this works, consider running with said baby in a running stroller so you both get some fresh air.
- Hail, tornado, ice storm, lightning, extreme heat, smoke due to fire. It's possible to run in rain, wind, snow, even mild hail. But weather conditions that can hurt—or kill—you should be avoided.
- Scary, dangerous darkness. Running predawn and post-sundown is both doable and energizing; it can make you feel like a rebel and a badass getting your sweat on as you run by people in their cozy houses. (And for more on how to run in the dark safely, see page 80.) But if you're in an area that is known to be unsafe, don't have anyone to run with, and/or just don't feel comfortable doing it and can't squeeze a run in during daylight, the treadmill is a safe and viable option.
- You're an occasional control freak. Sometimes, it can be fun to have your exact pace and distance beamed at you through an LED display on a treadmill console.
- You own one and can hop on it while your young kids are napping, while the aforementioned weather blows in, or when it's the middle of the night (or any time of day).

HOW TO FIND A TREADMILL

Mostly all gyms, aside from CrossFit "boxes," ninja warrior or parkour facilities, or your kids' gymnastics facility, have treadmills. So do hotel gyms.

HOW TO MAKE SURE YOU ENJOY IT

Professional runner, endurance coach, and race director Jacob Puzey set the world record for running fifty miles on a treadmill (4:57:45) in 2016. That means this guy ran almost five hours straight on a treadmill, not to mention the numerous hours he spent training on one. Puzey praises the merits of the machine, citing everything from time-saving, to working on form, to avoiding having to carry bear spray on a run if you live in bear country (which he does, in Canmore, Alberta, Canada).

And though he admits that treadmill running isn't as stimulating as running outdoors, there's an upside to that, too. "Being bored isn't necessarily a bad thing," he says, explaining that without all the stimulation and distractions of running outside, he can focus on what his body is doing and what different paces and efforts feel like, and he can process thoughts and be creative. "Sometimes it's nice to see where our thoughts will take us," he says.

Heed these tips from the record holder to assure a safe treadmill experience.

» **Ease into it.** Don't make your first treadmill run a long run, warns Puzey. Start with easy sessions and go from there.

» **Wear comfy shoes.** Puzey points out how treadmills are made of plastic and wood (underneath cushioned belts) and that wearing a comfortable, well-cushioned running shoe can help avoid impact injuries.[1]

» **Run in the middle of the belt** as opposed to the front or the back, says Puzey. Running at the front or back can affect your gait/stride.

> ### !!! WARNING !!!
> Do not try to do fancy tricks on a treadmill in hopes of going viral on a YouTube video. These are usually popular because the subjects go flying off the back of the moving treadmill belt and land on their faces. (Otherwise, they go flying because they increased their pace or incline too abruptly . . . so, make gradual adjustments.)

---

1   For more on running shoes, see Chapter 4. For more on impact injuries, see Chapter 7.

TREADMILL SURVIVAL GUIDE

If you're not up for seeing where boredom will let your mind roam, try these boredom-busting tricks:

- **Mix it up.** Once you get a few easy runs in on the treadmill to get used to the machine, try mixing up paces and inclines (gradually; see sidebar). And once you start adding speedwork into your running (see Chapters 6 and 10), know that doing so on a treadmill makes the time fly by.

- **Watch something.** Whether you binge on Netflix, time a treadmill run session with a televised sporting event, or catch up on the news or a thrilling game of JEOPARDY!, watching something and running on a treadmill can take away any guilt about watching the boob tube.

- **Tune in.** Listening to music while treadmill running really strikes the right note with some people (hardy har har). And listening to podcasts and audiobooks or taking professional development courses while running can be an enriching (and addicting) combination.

TRY IT ALL!

Even though figuring out which types of running location, environment, and scenario works best for you will help you find the love, it can be fun to try various options. Each will serve up different experiences, all with their own adventures . . .

Sucky thought zapped by this chapter:

"I never know when or where to go."

"It's boring."

CHOOSE YOUR OWN ADVENTURE (AND IT WON'T BE)

This chapter is different from other chapters in this book. YOU and YOU ALONE are in charge of what happens in this chapter. YOU must use all your personality traits that make you YOU, the ones you homed in on in the quiz on page xii. In this section, YOU will guide yourself through adventures that only YOU choose. But don't despair. At any time, YOU can go back and make another choice, alter the path of your story, and change its result. (And to avoid dying of boredom, YOU should occasionally make different choices.)

KEY NO. 3 TO MAKING RUNNING NOT SUCK: RUN SOMEWHERE INSPIRING

Figuring out the kind of terrain, setting, and scene that inspires you will actually make you *crave* runs, which will get you out the door and wanting to stay out longer.

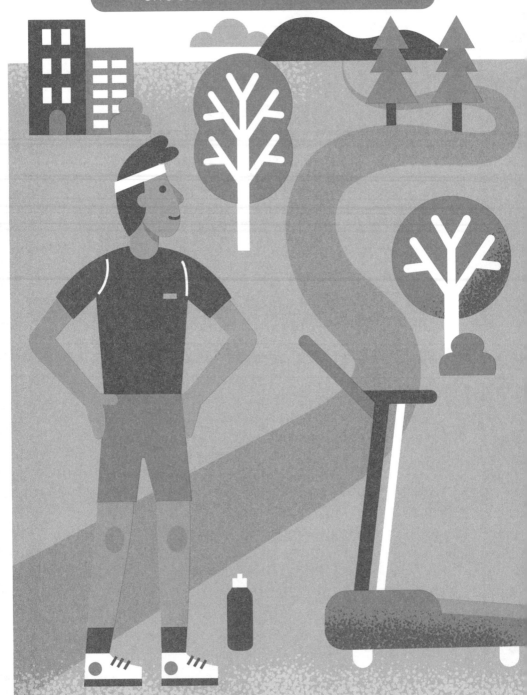

The goal is to figure out where you'll be most comfortable—and most inspired—to start off your run/walks. A lot of people say they hate running, but those same people only ever run on a treadmill or around a parking lot at their CrossFit gym in an all-out race. YOU are much more cunning than those people. YOU realize how much more enjoyable—and inspiring—it can be to run outside, somewhere pretty, with fresh air and things to look at, if that's what you choose. Every time you go out can be a new adventure, exploring your own neighborhood or a city park. (But if the thought of "exploring" gives you an anxiety attack, consider starting off on a track or even treadmill.)

First, YOU must choose the location of your run/walk. The choice YOU make will determine your experience. Try to choose wisely. GOOD LUCK!

· ·

You have grown into a human being who hates running. When you were a kid, you loved running. You are trying to figure out when and where you lost that feeling of joy when picking your feet up off the ground faster than a walking pace. Why is it that you now hate having both feet off the ground at the same time? No, you are not lazy. (Even if you are, you're not *all* the time.) Somewhere along the way since being a kid, you started hating running. Now you are on a mission to find the joy in it again.

You are in the right place. Use the knowledge you gleaned from Chapter 2 to figure out where—in what setting—you would most enjoy running (or run/walking, for starters). If you like breathing fresh air when you exercise, you have lots of options. In the great OUTDOORS, you can run on trails, dirt roads, paved paths, parks, ball fields, neighborhood streets, on beaches, or around a track. You'll be getting a healthy dose of oxygen, vitamin D, and the energy-boosting effects that studies have proven to trump running indoors. (Running outdoors has been proven to decrease tension, anger, and depression.)

If running outdoors gives you so much anxiety that you'd rather not run, it's okay to start running on a treadmill or on an indoor track. Running INDOORS can help build confidence and the desire you need to eventually head outside, and, as you learned in Chapter 2, has other merits.

You choose to run OUTDOORS. **Turn to page A.**

You choose to run INDOORS. **Turn to page B.**

OUTDOORS

Now that you have chosen to breathe fresh air, you look forward to all the added health benefits you'll be getting by running or run/walking outdoors. When you're outside, your mood improves (says science . . . and common sense). And when you're outside, you burn more calories and increase strength, as varied surfaces challenge your body differently from that of a treadmill. Plus, the varied surfaces and paces afforded by being outside can help mitigate overuse injuries you can get from running the same stride, over and over, on a treadmill.

And just think, when you're running outside, you get to look around at things like trees, clouds, and flowers. You get to see the world go by instead of staring at the back of some other gym-goer's sweaty head.

Now that you're committed to running outside most of the time (there is nothing wrong with the occasional indoor run), it's time to choose what type of outdoor running you want to do.

You can be more of the EXPLORING type and head out to find a neighborhood route, a paved path, or a dirt trail. Exploring can be highly motivating and help instill that sense of fun you once had playing capture the flag as a kid—and exploring can help you discover places within your city, town, or rural area you never knew existed before you were a runner.

Or you can choose to be a more of a CIRCULAR type of runner . . . at least at first, until you feel more comfortable about your running to venture out in one direction. If running in circles—either track-, small park-, or ball field–sized—sounds welcoming to you, you've got options. Also, if you are a very competitive person by nature, you may enjoy the measured, race-like environment of a track or other circular run where you can compare yourself to other people . . . or to yourself as you progress. This has been proven, anecdotally, to inspire competitive gym rat types to start running.

If you love the idea of EXPLORING and running somewhere other than around in circles,
turn to page C.

*If running in a CIRCULAR fashion sounds appealing—at least at first—***turn to page D.**

TREADMILL

Okay, you've chosen to start your running adventure on a TREADMILL. Unless you have a treadmill in your home, you'll be entering a gym near you. (FYI: Treadmills are super popular at gyms, so it's possible you'll need to sign up in advance—usually on a white board–type of signup sheet in the gym—for a time slot on the treadmill. And there may be maximum time limits in place so that gym-goers can share without getting in fights.)

When you step onto your treadmill, start by walking a few minutes to get used to the machine and settle into the motion while your body warms up. After five or ten minutes of walking, you can start your run intervals, the length of which you'll choose in Chapter 6.

While on the treadmill, you'll likely be surrounded by other people on treadmills. Try not to race them, at least until you've been running for a few months and have a solid base of running fitness.

You'll also likely be running in front of a television. Hopefully, the TV is playing something remotely interesting. Know that it can be tricky watching a TV and keeping your feet moving safely on a treadmill at the same time. You'll probably want to bring headphones for your treadmill run experience so you can tune in to what's on the TV, rock out to your own music, or learn something on a podcast or audiobook to help pass the time. Grab a towel from the gym's stash to wipe sweat from your eyes (wiping sweat on a loose-fitting shirt works, too, but can be more hazardous). Place the towel somewhere in front of you on the treadmill's console where it won't slip and fall onto the treadmill belt (no bueno). Be sure to bring a water bottle, which you can also place right on the console and have water within arm's reach.

Heads up, just in case you need to stop the belt, like, *now*: There's a stop button on all treadmills. There's also a red safety pull cord meant to be attached to your clothes, and if you haven't attached it to your clothes, pull it if you need the machine to stop for any reason.

You continue on this TREADMILLS-ONLY path if it feels right for you. Or maybe you're feeling a little bit more confident and want to venture outside, but really want to continue running in a controlled, measured environment like on an outdoor track.

You decide to stick to TREADMILLS ONLY. **Turn to page E.**

You decide you want to try running outside, but in a controlled, measured place. **Turn to page G.**

NEIGHBORHOOD

You have a little explorer in you . . . not an actual other person—this is not science fiction—but something within you likes the idea of exploring.

For starters, you'd like to explore your NEIGHBORHOOD. Starting a run from your doorstep is convenient (as is running home from your place of work, or someone else's neighborhood from a hotel while traveling). The best way to do this, of course, is to look at a map beforehand and plot a general course—nothing too complicated. You can also (especially if you live in a city or town with streets that run in a grid) head out the door without a set plan, but only make turns in one direction and end up right back at your doorstep. Or run in one direction for a set amount of time and return in the same direction, not making any turns in between. It's really hard to mess up a straight line.

But if and when that little explorer within you gets bigger, you'll start venturing farther out—and in more directions—in your neighborhood. When you do this, it's a good idea to carry a phone or watch with a mapping application (and the ability to call someone) in case you do get lost. It's also a good idea to have some money with you, in case you find yourself unexpectedly far from home and want to take public transportation, cab, or Uber or Lyft home.

To stay safe when crossing streets on these exploring runs in your neighborhood, be sure to abide by all pedestrian laws, including stopping at stoplights, crossing at crosswalks, and not jaywalking. If you're running around a blind corner, remember to cross the street where it's safe to do so and run on the other side of the street until it's safe to cross back over. Don't assume cars are going to stop; wait to be sure. It's always a good idea to make eye contact with the drivers of cars before you cross the street—that way, you know they see you before you step foot into the crosswalk.

When running on rural or city streets that don't have a sidewalk or dedicated pedestrian path, run on the side of the street that faces traffic. This is a safety measure: running toward traffic allows you to see cars approaching (rather than have them sneak up on you) so you can jump out of the way if a car is veering too close.

Now you need to decide if you're going to run the SAME NEIGHBORHOOD ROUTES all the time or if you'll further feed that inner EXPLORER.

*If you want to stay in your neighborhood and run the SAME NEIGHBORHOOD ROUTES over and over, **turn to page E.***

*If you want to get outside of your neighborhood and EXPLORE, **turn to page J.***

CIRCULAR

You like circles. Either that or you like the idea of running around a track, a ball field, a small park, or in laps around your neighborhood . . . and that is totally fine.

Running on a track can actually help certain people go from hating running to thinking it's not so bad. Those types of people include gym rats, competitively wired people, people who thrive on running short, fast intervals (maybe who played ball sports), and those intimidated by running anywhere else.

Maybe you fall into the first camp and love the measured, speed-oriented nature of a TRACK and perhaps the idea of comparing yourself to others within a social workout. A track might also just evoke the feeling of competition, even if the only thing you're racing is the clock. And if you've made your way to the track simply because you're intimidated by the thought of running anywhere else, you're in luck: it is virtually impossible to get lost on a track.

Maybe you want to run laps of some sort, but not at a track. You are also in luck, because there are options that maybe you've never thought of before.

*If you want to experience running on a TRACK, **turn to page F.***

*If you want to run in laps, but not on a track, **turn to page G.***

BOREDOM (DOOM)

You've chosen to stick to the same running experience every time you lace up. Unfortunately, this wasn't a wise choice, and your running has sadly died of boredom. (If you get another life, try mixing it up.)

The End. (Or is it?)

TRACK

First things first—find a running TRACK (hint: try a middle school, high school, or college; elementary schools are less likely to have them). Then save yourself some frustration and look up the times that you're allowed on that track (usually when school isn't in session, after practice times and on weekends, and outside of your region's outdoor track season). Good job! You're there by yourself, with a running partner, or with a group. Now what?

First of all, know that most people run counterclockwise around a track. So even if you're there by yourself, know that someone might show up to share the track with you, and it's a lot easier to share if you're both running in the same direction. (If you run on the track often, though, consider switching directions once in a while so you don't get overuse injuries from making only left turns. Just be aware and mindful of other runners, since you're going against the grain.)

Secondly, know that lane 1, the inside lane on the track, is the shortest distance around. If you're measuring your effort by time, not distance, consider running on the outside lanes. Once you start timing intervals—like how long it takes to run four hundred meters (a quarter mile, and once around a track)—you'll want to be in lane 1, if possible. (See Chapter 9 for track etiquette.)

With that squared away, start your workout by walking for five or ten minutes, as you should if you're running anywhere else. Then launch into whatever run or run/walk intervals you're there to do (plenty of those in Chapter 6).

If you choose to run on a TRACK, and only on a track, every time you head out, **turn to page E.***

If you like the idea of running in circles but want to have options beyond a track, **turn to page G.***

LAPS, BUT NOT A TRACK

You like circles but also squares, rectangles, and odd shapes. Running on BALL FIELDS, in PARKS, and in laps around your NEIGHBORHOOD all provide routes that give you the benefits of being outdoors, while minimizing the likelihood of getting lost and encountering unknowns.

On a ball field, you'll likely be running on grass, which is gentler on your joints than harder surfaces but can also be kind of unruly—long, uncut grass can feel cumbersome and draining to run through and can hide hazards like potholes and sprinklers.

Parks, both small and large, often have paved pedestrian paths *and* ribbons of dirt trails. Sometimes, they also have grassy ball fields.

If you want to run in a PARK or FIELD, **turn to page H.**

If you want to run NEIGHBORHOOD laps, **turn to page I.**

BALL FIELD

You've chosen to run laps around a grassy BALL FIELD. Safety Note: This is not ideal when a game of baseball is going on and it's a small field. (Foul ball! *Smack.*) However, during other sports—especially those of your group of carpool kids—or during no sports at all, grassy ball fields can be a great place to run.

Warm up by walking, as always, before starting to run. Be extra careful with your footing in tall grass; run with shorter strides than normal. It's a lot easier to recover from getting tripped up when your strides are short than it is when your strides are long. Otherwise, enjoy the ease on your joints provided by the grass. If you want to dabble in barefoot running, a grassy field is the perfect place to do it. Consider doing a few strides barefoot across the field at the end of your run, unless, of course, that means you'd be running straight through a peewee football game. (Or through a minefield of dog poop.)

Choose to only run on BALL FIELDS for the rest of your life? **Turn to page E.**

Want to run in circles on PAVEMENT? **Turn to page C.**

Want to run around a PARK or in another natural environment? **Turn to page I.**

PARK

Maybe you've found a PARK near your home or place of work. If it's a small park, you can run laps around it. If it's larger, you might be pleasantly surprised by the number of routes and paths winding throughout (think Central Park). Most parks have paved pedestrian paths, and many larger parks (think San Francisco's Golden Gate Park) have dirt trails winding throughout, often paralleling the paved or concrete routes. Safety Note: Be aware that trails that wind into dense brush in urban parks can lead to unwelcome surprises. Don't go it alone or in the dark if exploring said trails.

Parks can be entertaining and sometimes inspiring places to run, as other runners, Rollerbladers, fitness jugglers, slackliners, acroyogis, cyclists, and the like frequent parks to get their exercise on and enjoy the fresh air.

Parks also have things that can come in really handy to runners: bathrooms. And water fountains. But don't rely on the water fountains always working or bathrooms always being unlocked.

Decide to run in the same PARK, over and over, on the same route for the remainder of your days? **Turn to page E.**

The experience of running in a park have you itching to EXPLORE more? **Turn to page J.**

EXPLORE

You might get lucky and find some great route options by heading out the door of your home, office, or dorm room. But venturing farther from the doorstep can connect you to a whole new network of opportunity.

It's time to figure out surface and experience type for your exploring self.

If you answered *yes* to question number 6 on the quiz on page xii, then you're a nature lover. You love being outdoors, surrounded by trees, grass, dirt, and pretty things to look at.

If the idea of a trail freaks you out or you'd rather be amid nature without so much dirt, consider running on PAVED PATHS that can still serve up a good dose of the outdoors. These paths will let you run without having to stop at traffic lights, negotiate bike messengers, or dodge people with briefcases.

Running on TRAILS will give you constant variety. It will make you feel like you're on a mini-adventure every time you head out. Know that a "trail" doesn't have to mean a steep, rugged, rocky, narrow path straight up a mountain. A smooth, gentle dirt path is also a trail and can still give you an enjoyable sense of adventure.

If you like nature but prefer the notion of a PAVED PATH over dirt, **turn to page K.**

If you like the idea of running on dirt TRAILS, **turn to page L.**

PAVED PATHS

You've chosen to seek out PAVED PATHS. Good choice! Even major urban areas provide running and walking routes that are uninterrupted by cars, driveways, and stoplights, at least for the most part. (Think New York City's West Side Highway running path, for instance.)

Know that paved paths meant for pedestrians are usually parallel to paved paths meant for cyclists. Look for painted clues on the pavement: a painted bike means—no kidding!—it's a bike path. You want to run on the part where there's a painted pedestrian, and as far right as possible.

Though they're car-free, paved paths can be hazardous in other ways, so stay alert. Not everyone will know the paths are separate for bikers and foot travelers, so be aware of zooming bike commuters and fitness riders, as well as others on foot.

A benefit of running on a paved path in an urban area is that many have water fountains along the route, and some even have bathrooms. As an added bonus, they also often have mile markers and streetlights.

Choose to run out and back on the same PAVED PATH, day in and day out? **Turn to page E.**

Feel like exploring some DIRT? **Turn to page L.**

DIRT

You've decided to explore trails, which will amp up your dosage of a good old-fashioned nature immersion.

Not all trails are gnarly, cliff-hanging paths up Mount Everest. There are smooth dirt paths alongside rivers, grass fields, groves of trees, and pastures of cows and horses. These paths might convince you not only that running *doesn't suck* but also that you might *actually like it.*

In fact, even running on a DIRT ROAD in a rural environment can give you a trail-like running experience (and can be very convenient, if you live in that kind of environment).

And NARROW TRAILS, both mellow and gnarly, exist and can be a joy to run.

You like the idea of running on a rural, DIRT ROAD. **Turn to page M.**

You'd rather run a NARROW TRAIL, smooth or rugged. **Turn to page N.**

COUNTRY ROAD

You have access to a country road. The dirt surface is easier on your joints than concrete or pavement, and the uneven surface can strengthen all the small stabilizing muscles in your lower legs, all the way up to your core. (Just pay attention to your footing to avoid twisting an ankle.)

Your country road may take you home (to the place . . . where you belong), and/or it might lead you past cow pastures, farms, and other scenic and entertaining sights that can increase the enjoyment of your run. For safety purposes, when running on a dirt road—or a paved road, for that matter—run against traffic. This is especially important on roads where there isn't much shoulder and on roads where cars and trucks might not be used to seeing runners, like on most dirt roads. You want to be able to see cars approaching and hop off to the side if you need to. Just like running in a neighborhood, if there's a blind corner, you'll want to cross the road when it's safe and run on the opposite side—where cars can see you—before switching back to the side where you'll be facing traffic.

Now you need to decide if you're going to stick to running this COUNTRY ROAD all the time or if you want to experience any other kind of running, including TRAILS.

If you choose to run the same COUNTRY ROAD, out and back, over and over, yup, you guessed it . . . **turn to page E.**

If the idea of running TRAILS sounds appealing, **turn to page N.**

SMOOTH TRAILS

Not all trails are gnarly. And not all trails even require trail running–specific shoes. Not only does trail running allow you to run amid nature, but the hard-packed dirt that makes up most running trails is easier on your joints than pavement or concrete. You might find you love running on a natural surface, perhaps next to a babbling creek or alongside tall grasses and trees. (To find trails like this, check out page 24.)

Smooth trails can be wide or narrow. If they're wide, you can run side by side with a running buddy. If you're sharing the trail with bikes, other runners, joggers, or groups of kids in a summer camp, be ready to change formation and run single file to help keep the peace on the trail. And if you need to pass any of the above groups (and good on you if you're passing a bike), then try coughing or saying, "Excuse me" or "Hi." You can also say, "On your left," but refrain from yelling this with an irritable tone in your voice, lest you sound like a self-important maniac.

If you discover you love running on this type of surface, you can now decide if you'll keep running on this type of trail all the time (but not the same exact location, or you're bound to suffer the consequences on page E) or experience a more RUGGED TRAIL.

To avoid dying of boredom, you decide to try other running scenarios.
Turn to pages B, C, D, F, G, H, I, J, K, L, M, and P.

You like the idea of running a more RUGGED TRAIL. **Turn to page O.**

RUGGED TRAILS

Single-track trails (wide enough for a single user, not two side by side) that wind through wilderness—urban, mountainous, rural, or wherever—offer a great sense of adventure and potential for fun. These types of trails can be smooth or riddled with rocks, roots, ruts, and the like. That bumpy ride can make you feel kid-like, hopping between obstacles (don't touch the hot lava!) and negotiating the terrain like a ninja. Those same obstacles build lower leg strength, balance, and core strength . . . but they can also make you fall on your face (which, if you think about it, is also kid-like), so pay attention to where you're going.

To build up strength and balance that can help prepare you to negotiate terrain like this so you *don't* fall on your face, turn to page 9. And to use your resourcefulness in finding a trail like this, turn to page 24.

Running on a single-track trail—smooth or not—will give you all those great benefits of being in nature and coerces you to be present during your run. This can be a healthy respite for people suffering from anxiety or general stress during their regular lives. Being fully present as you negotiate a narrow trail and rocks and other obstacles forces you to be mindful for that period of time. (Concentrate or wipe out.) See page 6 for more on mindful running.

On a single-track trail, it's best to focus fully on your surroundings. Not only is it a joy to hear the sounds of nature, but not wearing headphones will allow you to be aware of potential dangers—anything from fast-approaching humans who want to pass by you to, say, a growling or rattling sound coming from the bushes (in which case, you should back away and change directions).

And on a trail, you'll want to either know where you're going or run with a friend who knows where he or she is going. Getting majorly lost *can* be kind of fun, but exposing yourself to a full day of dangers isn't healthy for your loved ones (or you, unless you're Bear Grylls).

Now that you enjoy trails, and you know better than to run the same trail all the time (and avoid suffering the fate on page E!), you can decide to mix it up.

*You wisely choose to mix up your running, so **turn to pages B, C, D, F, G, H, I, J, K, L, M, N, and P.***

Running on a BEACH sounds nice, and you either live near one or are traveling to one.
Turn to page P.

BEACH

Ah, the beach. What a lovely place to be. The beach can be a great place to run, or it can be a total ass-kicker.

First things first: not all beaches are ideal for running. Loose, dry sand or short, steep shores will absorb your energy and make your run so challenging that it could be miserable, unless you're a seasoned runner looking to mix things up.

Beaches with wide, flat (or at least semi-flat), hard-packed sand when the tide is low can feel downright springy underfoot, and are better for running than rocky shores or deep-sand, energy-sucking beaches. But even on hard-packed sand, your feet and lower legs will still be working a little harder than they do on hard surfaces like concrete. Therefore, it's a good idea to adjust your runs to be shorter than normal when at the beach, at least until you build up strength and endurance for this specific terrain.

Some beaches have very slanted shorelines, which can wreak havoc on knees and other joints and the muscles connected to them. Be sure to run in both directions (an out-and-back approach is great for beach runs, instead of running out on the beach and back on the road) to ensure you're not putting more strain on one side of the body than the other.

If you're an experienced runner, consider a short, deep-sand run for a super-intense (read: time-efficient!) workout. But beware: this takes a ton of effort due to the stabilizing your muscles need to do, so you might tire out much more quickly than you do normally.

And it is highly advised to splash some ocean or lake water on your face when you're done with your run. Or better yet, jump in!

Go back to discover what to expect in any scenario you haven't yet explored.

Or turn the page to move on, now that you're fully informed on your options.

And if you've died from the fate on page E, you can now come back to life and turn the page.

Congratulations!

You've discovered all the different environments for running and are now equipped to choose your own adventure every time you head out for a run.

Sucky thought zapped by this chapter:
"Running is boring."

"All that stuff."

HOME IN ON THE GEAR YOU REALLY NEED

All you really need to go running is this:

Yes, you could run in what you're wearing right now—just think about the people who are late for a bus or who encounter a wild dog while carrying a steak. You could run totally naked. People do that on purpose, actually. It's a thing. But any clothes, shoes, accessories, or gadgets you might buy that are specifically designed for running have the potential to do two things: 1) motivate you to get out and use them; 2) make running suck a lot less.

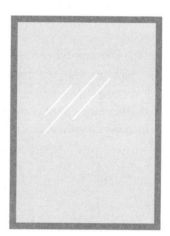

Pretend this is a mirror.[1]

Most pieces of new running gear will do #1. Not nearly every piece of running gear does #2. (Imagine a new shirt chafing you to shreds with every arm swing.) This chapter will teach you how to be a discerning shopper to pinpoint what gear actually enhances a run so you enjoy it, which can add longevity to the motivation factor. Win-win!

---

1 Publisher did not want to pay for reflective paper.

KEY NO. 4 TO MAKING RUNNING NOT SUCK: BUY GREAT GEAR

While all you need to run is you, there's something extremely motivating about new gear. And while buying anything new can motivate you to try it out for one run, buying something new and really great will motivate you over and over. The key is educating yourself on what makes great gear great (by reading this chapter) and then making a purchase or two.

In a 2012 study in the *Journal of Experimental Psychology*, researchers coined the term "enclothed cognition" in order to "describe the systematic influence clothes have on the wearer's psychological processes." The study found that when people put on a lab coat (which makes them think of a doctor), their attention increases.

The takeaway? If you put on new running clothes, you'll feel more like a runner and might feel more motivated to hit the road, trails, or treadmill. And if you put on new running gear of any sort—shoes, socks, GPS tracker, skin lubrication—that makes your run more enjoyable. It also probably means your running frequency will continue in an upward pattern:

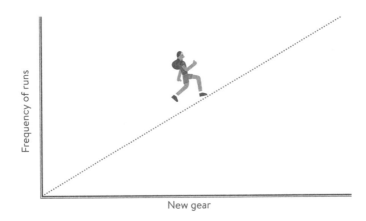

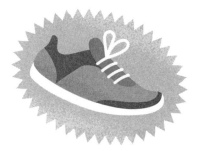

THE ALMIGHTY RUNNING SHOE

There is no shortage of running shoes that promise to make you *faster, more comfortable, more sure-footed, able to run a hundred miles, able to run until you're a hundred years old, able to fly, run more naturally, run more like a hunter-gatherer.* But no matter what promises a shoe company might be making, the most important thing is that you need to be fitted for the right pair for *you.* Every pair of feet is different, and every person runs differently. There is no magic bullet brand or specific shoe model that works for everyone.

Also, if you've been running in your mom's old shoes, your checkered Vans, your hiking boots, two-year-old shoes, your wife's shoes, five-year-old shoes, your Zumba shoes, ten-year-old shoes, or shoes you've worn to your nursing job every day . . . there's no wonder why you think running sucks.

Running does suck in old shoes or shoes that aren't right for your foot, your body, or your style of running.

HOW TO FIND THE SHOE THAT'S RIGHT FOR YOU

It is highly recommended that you start your search for new running shoes at a specialty running store. Sure, you can find every shoe in those stores online, but specialty running shoe store employees are trained to help you find the perfect pair of running shoes for your body, running habits, and goals. They'll ask you questions about the kind of running you're looking to do (Hint: You answered some of those questions for yourself in the Know-Thyself-to-Become-a-Runner Quiz); they'll measure and look at your feet (Wide or narrow? Bunions or insanely long toes?) and inspect the bottoms of the shoes you wear on a day-to-day basis to assess the wear-pattern. (Inside/medial[1] side of the outsole worn down? You need some medial support.) What they won't do: roll their eyes when you say you like the blue shoe on the wall and the one with the cool pattern. They're trained to listen to your likes and then go to the back room and pull out those shoes and a bunch of other ones they think would work (probably better) for you.

GAIT ANALYSIS: WHAT AND WHY

Your friendly shoe salesperson may have you run on a treadmill for a gait analysis. They'll put you in different shoes and watch you run by studying—possibly by videotaping—how your feet strike the treadmill, if your hips are out of whack when you run, and other gait traits. They'll assess how different shoes affect these factors, then help fit you with the shoe that helps guide you into, hopefully, the most natural, comfortable, and efficient running stride possible.

Your helpful salesperson may then start throwing out a bunch of technical running shoe terms. See the "Running Shoe Term Glossary" for a cheat sheet to figure out what on earth they're talking about.

RUNNING SHOE TERM GLOSSARY

Note: You do *not* need to know these terms, and your salesperson can explain them, but if you're curious (or really insistent on shopping online for shoes yourself and come across these terms), here they are, defined:

SHOE PARTS AND CHARACTERISTICS

» **Upper:** The part of the shoe that encapsulates your foot, made of mesh or other synthetic material. Basically, everything up from the midsole.

» **Midsole:** The foam cushy stuff between the outsole and the upper/footbed.

---

1 See glossary.

» **Cushioning:** What the midsole is mostly there for; also found in the tongue and around the heel collar for comfort.

» **Outsole:** The underbelly of the shoe. The part that touches the ground.

» **Tread:** The patterned rubber on the outsole.

» **Laces:** The . . . laces.

» **Eyelets:** The little holes that the laces poke through that help adjust volume fit.

» **Volume fit:** How loose or snug the shoe feels around your foot (as opposed to how long or short the shoe is in length).

» **Tongue:** The thing that looks like a tongue that lies flat against the top of your foot, beneath the laces.

» **Heel collar:** The opening around the heel that encircles your ankle. Where you step into the shoe.

» **Heel counter:** The curved piece that fits around your heel, more rigid than the rest of the upper.

» **Last:** The shape of the interior of the shoe that affects how the shoe fits your foot.

» **Forefoot:** The interior of the shoe where the front of your foot (the ball of your foot and toes) sits.

» **Medial:** The side of the shoe that faces your opposite foot.

» **Lateral:** The side of the shoe that faces outward and away from your body.

» **Flex:** How bendy the shoe is.

» **Flex grooves:** Cuts made in the outsole to make a shoe more bendy.

» **Torsional rigidity:** How un-bendy a shoe is when twisted.

» **Insole:** The most-often removable piece of material—shaped like the bottom of your foot—which sits in your shoe and offers cushion. Also referred to as **footbed** (picture your foot resting comfortably here).

» **Toe bumper:** Additional rubber on the front of a trail shoe meant to protect your toes from getting stubbed.

RUNNER CHARACTERISTICS ADDRESSED BY DIFFERENT TYPES OF SHOES

» **Pronation:** When feet roll in toward the medial side.

» **Flat-footed:** A foot that doesn't have a high arch, often causing pronation.

» **Supination:** When feet roll out toward the lateral side. (Rarer than pronation.)

» **Heel striker:** A runner who lands on their heel first with every step. (Most humans are heel strikers.)

» **Midfoot striker:** A runner who lands on their midfoot first with every step. (Known as efficient runners.)

» **Forefoot striker:** A runner who lands on their forefoot first with every step. (Only sprinters, really.)

HAVING TO DO WITH HOW SHOES ARE MADE

» **Stability/motion-control:** Characteristic in certain shoes that is meant to correct pronation/motion by your foot that could cause injury.

» **Neutral:** Shoes with less structure that don't correct pronation or supination.

» **Light stability:** A touch of stability for people who only pronate a little.

» **Stack height:** Refers to how high off the ground the foot sits, usually given in two measurements: one for the heel, and one for the forefoot. And they're usually different, with the heel sitting higher off the ground (on top of more cushioning) than the forefoot.

» **Offset:** The difference in stack heights between the heel and the forefoot.

» **Zero drop:** When the stack height of the heel and the forefoot are the same, the shoe has "zero drop" from heel to forefoot. Meant to mimic "natural" running, as our bare feet have zero drop from heel to forefoot.

» **Maximal:** A term coined for maximally cushioned shoes—you know, the ones that sorta look like moon shoes but also look really comfortable.

» **Minimal:** A term coined for shoes with minimal cushioning and minimal structure, meant to closely mimic running without any shoes on at all for a "natural" running experience.

MORE THAN IF THE SHOE FITS . . .

"A lot of factors go into fitting someone with the right running shoe specific to them," says Mark Plaatjes, owner of In Motion Running in Boulder, Colorado, physical therapist, and past world-champion marathoner. "Each individual runner's mechanics, how they move, how they run, where they run, their foot shape, how the surface of their foot interacts with the interior of a shoe all adds up to proper options for that particular runner. That's why it's worth going to a good specialty running store."

TRAIL SHOE VS. ROAD SHOE VS. HYBRID VS. RACING FLAT

» **Road shoe:** A shoe made specifically for running on concrete and asphalt, most often more flexible and with much less traction underfoot than a trail shoe. Road shoes can work on trails but can feel slippery and flimsy on dirt. They range from beefy stability/motion-control models to maximally cushioned bounce-mobiles to skimpy, lightweight racing flats.

» **Trail shoe:** A shoe made specifically for running trails, with a more durable, protective upper and more aggressive tread than a road shoe, as well as other trail-friendly features like durable, uppers and toe bumpers. Trail shoes can work on roads but can feel clunky and stiff on non-trail surfaces where such traction isn't really necessary.

» **Hybrid road/trail shoe:** A shoe that runs well on both roads and trails, often with a touch of traction underfoot and moderate flexibility. Hybrid shoes aren't necessarily meant to excel on either road or trail—they can feel slippy on steep, rugged trails and clunkier on paved surfaces than shoes built specifically for roads.

» **Racing flat:** A shoe that is built to be extremely lightweight and minimal so its wearer can fly around tracks and in races. Not meant to be comfortable for pounding miles at leisurely speeds. Racing flats are super flexible, not at all supportive, and have very minimal cushioning. But, man, are they lightweight.

HOW TO WASH (AND NOT RUIN) YOUR RUNNING SHOES

It is really tempting to throw a pair of dirty, smelly running shoes into a washing machine, but don't do it. The deep, extended soak combined with the sloshing and spinning of your machine can warp or otherwise ruin your shoes. What's worse than washing, however, is drying. Heat can melt the glues manufacturers use to keep shoe parts together, causing the shoes to fall apart. To safely clean your dirty, stinky shoes, do the following:

1. If slightly dirty, take a soft-bristled brush, like an old toothbrush, dipped in gentle dishwashing soap or detergent and scrub off the dirt.

2. If very dirty, take a garden hose and spray down shoes (concentrating on the exterior and avoiding the interior of the shoe, if possible), then rub with a soft-bristled brush dipped in gentle dishwashing soap or detergent. If shoes are muddy, either clean immediately, or let dry and bang together to get the bulk of the caked-on stuff off before cleaning any residual mud.

3. Rinse with cool water, either by spraying or spot-rinsing with a wet rag. Don't dunk 'em.

4. Shake off as much water as possible, then loosen the laces, remove the insoles to dry separately, and stuff the interior with newspapers to help absorb moisture. Set out to dry, but keep them out of direct sunlight (which has the same effect as a hot clothes dryer).

5. To combat odor, try potpourri-like products that stash inside shoes when they're not on feet.

RUNNING GEAR: THE NON-SHOE STUFF

Running gear encompasses everything from socks to phone-holding contraptions, shorts to hairbands, sunglasses to sports bras. While you don't desperately *need* all the things, having some key items can ease you into less sucky running, which is kind of priceless.

APPAREL (A.K.A. CLOTHES)

Running clothes differ from regular clothes in that they're made out of materials that don't soak through with sweat and hold moisture (cotton kills!). Most any running apparel worth its salt is made of sweat-wicking synthetic fabric of some sort meant to pull sweat from your body to the exterior of the fabric and evaporate it into the atmosphere so you dry quickly. (There are some cotton/synthetic blends that won't kill you.) Technical wool running apparel pulls sweat from your body, and while it does stay slightly wet, it helps to regulate your body temperature.

Running gear is also different from, say, your tutu because of streamlined fits that won't get in your way when you run. Features like smooth, flat seams, and zippers that are positioned so they won't chafe the shit out of your skin with every step and arm swing help.

And then there are run-friendly features in apparel, like small pockets to hold your keys, ventilation panels to help you keep your cool, moisture-blocking-yet-breathable jackets to protect you in foul weather, and the like.

COVER YOUR: BUTT

» **Shorts:** Not all running shorts have to be bare-almost-everything tiny. Shorts come in lengths from a little cheeky to basketball player–long and everything in between. And while some runners prefer short shorts so they're completely unrestricted, well-made long shorts (lightweight, airy material, good fit) shouldn't inhibit your stride too much. Short shorts don't have to be the ass cheek–baring split shorts you see on elite runners; they can simply have a short inseam to keep them out of your way. Short shorts should have flat or smooth seams around the leg openings so they don't rub or chafe your inner thighs.

» **Compression shorts:** While some are actual medical-grade compression for blood flow, either throughout or in panels, skin-hugging shorts worn by men and women are often referred to as "compression" shorts. These come in many different inseams, from short-short (often referred to as "booty shorts" or "hot pants") to mid-thigh, and the benefit is that no material rubs your skin or flaps in the wind. Benefits of actual compression include support and increased circulation.

» **Skirts:** Running skirts, most with compression shorts or brief underwear built in, offer a nifty little combo: close-fitting material directly against the leg, but with a bit more modesty (no bum outlines) in what can be a more flattering silhouette. They also can be cool in summer months (think Marilyn Monroe on the subway grate).

» **Tights:** Tights are, well, tight, and therefore don't allow much airflow to touch your skin—a good thing in cold weather. They're also one of the best options for avoiding chafing, since they prevent skin-on-skin contact. Tights come in a range of fabric thickness feels, and fanciness. Seeking muscle support? Shop for compression panels or 100-percent compression (though get ready to be squeezed). Seeking extra ventilation and/or trendy styling? Shop for options with mesh paneling. Live in a frozen tundra and need armor from the wicked winter wind? Shop for tights with wind-blocking material on the fronts combined with more breathable backsides.

» **Capris:** Capris are tights knocked off at the mid-calf, and they offer seasonal versatility, as they're warmer than shorts and cooler than full-length tights. These also come in fancy fabrics, minus the wind-blocking winter armor.

» **Pants:** Running pants are loose-fitting tights, some with roomier thigh areas and tapered ankles (think of the classic track pant silhouette), some with straight legs. Like tights, pants come in a range of fabrics and weights.

» **Underwear:** You may or may not prefer to wear underwear beneath your running bottoms (though they're not necessary under running shorts that come with briefs built in). If you do, choose well-fitting underwear made out of sweat-wicking material. No one wants baggy, soggy underwear (while running or, well, ever). Running-specific underwear is constructed to be both well-fitting and sweat-wicking.

HOW TO WASH (AND NOT RUIN) YOUR RUNNING CLOTHES

Since you spent your hard-earned money on fancy running clothes, it's worth taking care of them. Here's how to extend the life of running apparel made of technical fabrics:

COLD WATER AND REGULAR DETERGENT. You don't need to handwash everything, but use cold water in your laundry machine. Regular cycle is fine; gentle cycle is safest. And regular detergent is fine, while sport-specific laundering soap is safest.

AIR-DRY IF POSSIBLE. Air-drying is the safest way to dry and extend the life of running gear, since the heat from a dryer can break down synthetic fibers, which means your tights will be less tight over time. If you need to machine dry, select a low-heat setting.

TIPS FOR BUYING BOTTOMS

» **Try them on:** Try on different cuts and styles to see what you feel the most comfortable and confident in. Forcing yourself to wear booty compression shorts that make you self-conscious will not motivate you to run. Looking forward to wearing your running skirt (or booty compression shorts, if that's your thing) will.

» **Assess comfort:** Aside from the emotional comfort above, assess if anything about the bottoms is physically uncomfortable. A seam that rubs you the wrong way in the dressing room will annoy thehell out of you on—and likely totally ruin—a run.

» **Think about your needs:** Need a secure pocket for your house key or car key? Most running bottoms have a key pocket, but make sure. If you're running at dusk, dawn, or in the dark, make sure what you buy has reflective details.

COVER YOUR: BELLY

» **Singlet:** Nothing says running nerd more than a singlet. Thin-strapped and revealing (but light, airy, and speed-inspiring), professional runners often rock singlets, and you can, too, if you feel so inclined.

» **Tank:** Wider-strapped than a singlet, a tank made specifically for running can be a godsend in warm temps.

» **Short-sleeve T-shirt:** Running T-shirts come in tight-fitting, loose-fitting, and all sorts of styles. Some even double as casual wear.

» **Long-sleeve T-shirt:** Ditto on the above.

TIPS FOR BUYING SHIRTS

» **Try it on:** Same rule here as for bottoms: If it makes you feel confident and excited to wear it, it'll help get you running more often. If it doesn't, don't buy it, even if it's on sale for 90 percent off.

» **Swing your arms:** To test the chafe-ability, swing your arms back and forth to see if any material or seams annoy your inner arms. If it does, or they do, don't buy it.

» **Think about your needs:** If you're only buying one running shirt, a short-sleeve running T-shirt is the most versatile across the most weather situations. And consider reflective details for low-light running.

COVER (AND SUPPORT) YOUR: BOOBS[2]

» **Sports bra:** Ladies, if you're going to invest in one piece of running gear aside from a pair of shoes, it should be a good sports bra (or a few). Keep those things from bouncing on your run, or end up being both uncomfortable and uncomfortably stared at. And while studies haven't proven that supportive sports bras actually spare the Cooper's ligaments that hold on to your breast tissue, if there's a chance it'll help . . .

   » Plus, women runners with larger breasts can be pulled out of proper postural alignment when not wearing a supportive bra, which can wreak havoc on your body overall.

» **Shimmel:** A sports bra that extends down your torso like a tight-fitting tank top with a sports bra built in.

TIPS FOR BUYING SPORTS BRAS

» **Try it on:** A proper fit on a sports bra is paramount—too big and it won't do its job; too small and it'll make for a super-uncomfortable run. Most come in small, medium, large, XL, and sometimes XXL but some come in band and cup sizes (i.e., 32A or 38D). Dialing in the right fit will make a difference in your comfort.

» **Do a bounce test:** In the fitting room, jump up and down to test comfort and support.

» **Think about your needs:** Do you need the sports bra to be cute? Or will it be hiding underneath a tee? Want an imaginative place to stash a gel or key? Some sports bras have a pocket or pockets on the back or between the breasts.

---

2 Are you a dude who flipped to this page for some titillation? Get lost!

HOW TO TAKE OFF A SPORTS BRA IN PUBLIC

Changing out of a sweaty sports bra in public can be done, and it can come in really handy. (Nothing makes you colder and more uncomfortable than a sweaty sports bra long after your run.) Here's a how-to guide that can be done in a car, behind a tree, or wherever you're slightly hidden but not totally out of view:

1. Pull on a T-shirt or loose-fitting sweatshirt over said sweaty sports bra.
2. Pull one arm inside the shirt's arm hole, then pull that arm through the sports bra opening on that same side, using your opposite hand to pull the bra loose enough.
3. Pull that stinky, sweaty sports bra over your head toward the arm that's still trapped, and stick your free arm back out through the T-shirt hole.
4. Reach across your body and pull that sweaty thing right out the arm of the opposite T-shirt hole. Keeping arms inside your shirt, pull on a regular bra or go back through the top of your shirt to put on a dry sports bra (much more difficult) by first pulling it over your head, then by shoving one arm through at a time. Voilà!

COVER: IT ALL (OUTERWEAR)

» **Vest:** A vest made for running offers wind protection and a layer of warmth for your core, which can help keep you toasty without bulk. The downside is that a vest is hard to shed when you warm up (lack of sleeves means it can't be tied around your waist).

» **Jacket:** Running-specific jackets are categorized by what they're meant to block. Wind shells block wind and are often labeled as "water-resistant," which means they don't stop rain or snow from permeating the fabric but can hold off some moisture for a short amount of time.

- **Water-resistant jackets.** These block some moisture but aren't as bulletproof as fully waterproof jackets. They work well to block wind.
- **Waterproof jackets.** These are meant to block all rain and snow, and some breathe better than others. Look for breathable fabrics or ventilating features like holes in the armpits. Also known as hard-shell jackets.
- **Soft-shell jackets.** These are made of air-permeable, sometimes waterproof but at least water-resistant materials that breathe better than hard-shells (think sweatshirt versus trash bag). They're often thicker and therefore warmer than wind-/hard-shells, so they're best suited for cold (or cold and snowy) climates.
- **Hood vs. no hood.** A hood on a running jacket can do two things: 1) protect your head from the wind/rain/snow/cold; 2) drive you totally insane by flopping on the back of your neck when not in use. If you like the idea of a hood, make sure it doesn't flop too much (material and cut will affect this) by doing a bounce test, and check if it has a way to roll down and snap away, as some jackets do.

TIPS FOR BUYING JACKETS

» **Try it on:** It's true that sometimes buying something online, sight unseen, is cheaper and a lot easier. If you do that, make sure you read up on the different types of jackets (see the previous section) and read the features or specifications list about the jacket thoroughly. But if you can try on a jacket in the store, do it.

» **Swing your arms:** Do this to see if it either chafes or rubs, or if the fabric swish-swishes so noisily that it would annoy you on the run.

» **Think about your needs:** What weather situations will you most often be running in? Do you want a hood or not? Do you want to be able to tie it around your waist when not in use? (If so, try doing so in the store and jump around to see if it stays put.)

COVER YOUR: FEET (SOCKS)

» **No-show:** These are those tiny little socks that don't show when you're wearing shoes. They're great for summer running. Hazard: Dirt, tiny pebbles, and other extraneous items can sneak in between your feet and your socks and cause irritation, and if they don't stay up properly, you run the risk of developing a blister (which will definitely make your run suck).

» **Low-cut:** These socks can be seen peeking out the tops of most shoes and can help ward off abrasion from the heel collar or tongue of a running shoe. Hazard: Same as with no-show . . . gunk can sneak in and be buggin'.

» **Mid-cut:** Mid-cut socks extend past your ankle bone and can be great protection from trail gunk on off-road runs. Hazard: Funky tan lines.

» **Long:** Socks that extend over the calf aren't always made of compression material. Sometimes they're made of brightly colored or patterned sweat-wicking material and worn just for fun. Hazard: Funkier tan lines.

» **Compression.** Compression socks most often extend to the knee but also come in shorter lengths. The jury is out on their effectiveness, but people wear them to increase circulation (which aids recovery), support muscles due to the increased pressure, reduce swelling, and more. The key with compression socks (and other compression apparel pieces) is to make sure they're tight enough. If you want to give them a try, be sure to check with manufacturers and take your measurements. Hazard: Being stared at; denting your bank account.

WHY YOU NEED *RUNNING* SOCKS

Wearing cotton socks is like begging for a blister. Socks made for running are constructed out of sweat-wicking fabric and molded carefully to provide a secure, non-bunching, and non-irritating fit around your feet. Bottom line: They're worth it.

WHETHER THE WEATHER IS...

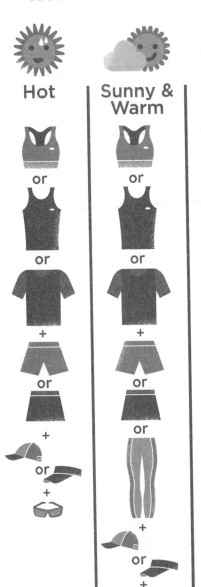

Hot

Sunny &
Warm

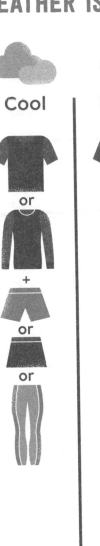

Cool

Rainy

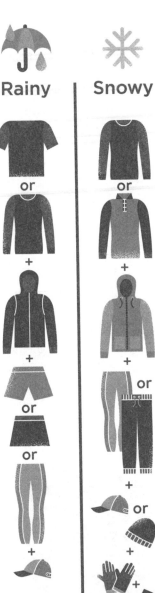

Snowy

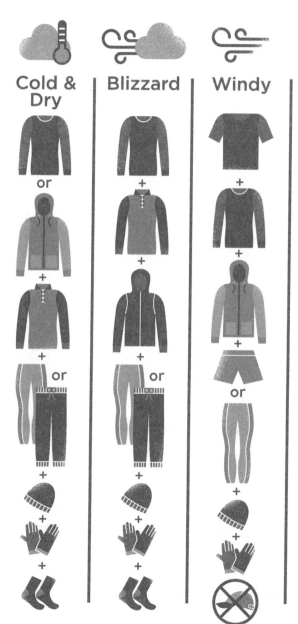

Cold & Dry

Blizzard

Windy

Trail

Weather dependent

AUXILIARY ELEMENTS

A whole slew of gadgets, gizmos, contraptions, and accessories exist under the umbrella of "running gear." Here's boiled-down information to help you navigate through them.

GADGETS

SIMPLE WATCHES — $

Tell time. Have chrono setting to easily time runs and run/walk intervals. Also have handy things like alarms.

WRIST COMPUTERS — $$-$$$

Most likely GPS-enabled to give you your pace and distance both while you're running and after (synching up to tracking software on your phone or computer that shows your route and works with social media apps). Some give you heart rate readings and other data like VO_2 max readings.

FITNESS TRACKERS WITHOUT GPS — $

Count steps and estimate distance, but aren't as accurate as a GPS watch or phone with GPS. Less expensive and simpler to use than those with GPS.

FITNESS TRACKERS WITH GPS — $$-$$$

Count steps, estimate distance, and offer colorful screens, maps, and pace tracking. More expensive than those without GPS.

SMARTWATCHES — $$$-$$$$

GPS-enabled smartwatches will give you your pace and distance and include features ranging from weather info to cell service. They'll also buzz, sometimes incessantly, with notifications from your phone (unless you change the settings).

SMARTPHONES — $$-$$$

Yes, smartphones tell time and track pace and time with certain apps, but they're hard to view mid-run (see next section).

PHONE-CARRYING CONTRAPTIONS

Running with a phone in your hand can be done, but so can dropping a phone you're carrying in your hand. Plus, many less-cumbersome solutions exist, such as waist-mounted belts that don't bounce too much, armbands, and even some handheld water bottle carriers with pockets large enough for a smartphone.

SUNGLASSES

Sunglasses shield your eyes from that fireball in the sky and reduce eye fatigue, which is great, since your body will be working hard enough on a run. Good running sunglasses will have:

- **Decent lenses:** Polarized or simple UV-blocking; photochromic that change with light conditions; or swap-out lenses for different light conditions.
- **Minimal movement:** They should stay in place on your face without slipping when you're sweaty, and they shouldn't bounce up and down on your nose bridge.
- **Zero fogging:** Avoid running in "fashion" glasses with giant, buglike lenses for this reason.

GLOVES/MITTENS

Gloves can offer an insane (in a good way) amount of warmth from fall to spring, which includes all the way through winter. And gloves come in a range of thicknesses and materials, from super-thin to winter weatherproof. Decide what your main needs are for gloves: Provide warmth on cool runs? Thin gloves made of sweat-wicking material will do. Keep your fingers from getting frostbite? Shop for windproof, slightly insulated (but still breathable) gloves. Need hand protection through a Minnesota winter? Buy insulated, weatherproof mittens. Mittens are warmer than gloves due to the warmth your fingers lend to each other.

HATS

Hats can be saviors on runs—they can shield you from the sun on a brutally hot day, keep rain out of your eyes in a downpour, or help you keep in some heat on a chilly day. Choose among the following for your climate, the weather, and the time of day:

» **Visor:** Benefit: Shields sun from eyes and face while letting your head breathe. Can keep sweat from dripping down from your head and onto your face and into your eyes. Look for: Quick-drying, lightweight, synthetic material (breathable mesh is a bonus); sweat-wicking panel at the forehead; adjustability in the back (unless it fits you perfectly).

» **Ball cap:** Benefit: Shields sun from eyes, face, and head, and protects from rain. Shields a bald head from sunburn and all scalps from sun damage. Can abate sweat (see visor). Look for: Quick-drying, lightweight, synthetic material (breathable mesh is a bonus); sweat-wicking panel at the forehead; adjustability in the back (unless it fits you perfectly).

» **Trucker hat:** Benefit: Shields sun from eyes, face, and head, protects from rain, and is trendy. Breathes well because of nylon, open mesh backside. Look for: Quick-drying, lightweight, synthetic material (breathable mesh is a bonus); sweat-wicking panel at the forehead; adjustability in the back (unless it fits you perfectly).

» **Beanie:** Benefit: Keeps your head warm, which can do a lot for keeping your whole body warm. Easy to stash away when you get too warm. Look for: Quick-drying, lightweight, thin synthetic material; packability (can you shove it in a pocket or pack when not in use on longer outings?).

» **Buff/Tuke:** Benefit: Keeps your head, neck, or face warm, which can do a lot for keeping your whole body warm. Easy to stash away when you get too toasty—you can wrap it around your wrist as a sweatband when not in use on your head or neck. Look for: Quick-drying, lightweight, thin synthetic material; packability (can you shove it in a pocket or pack when not in use on longer outings?).

HYDRATION SYSTEMS

Keep in mind that you don't really need one of these things until you're running around forty-five minutes or more at a time, unless it's midday in Florida in July. But here's the lowdown on your options for when you do want to carry water or energy fluids with you on the run.

» **Handheld:** Everything from four-ounce (half-cup) flasks up to twenty-ounce (two-and-a-half-cup) bottles contained within sweat-wicking material and comfortable straps that wrap around your hand. Generally speaking, the smaller the bottle/flask, the more comfortable it is to carry (and know that a regular shot of booze is one and a half ounces, for reference). Soft flasks collapse as you drink the fluids and they become empty, and hard flasks are easier to clean. If you carry a large-volume bottle, it's important to change hands every once in a while so you don't develop strange pains and/or lopsided biceps muscles.

» **Waist-mounted:** Waist-mounted packs made of sweat-wicking material carry everything from one to multiple four-ounce bottles, to larger bottles and flasks. Make sure you do the bounce test when shopping for a waist-mounted pack. Tip: Some find wearing them around the hips, instead of the waist, can keep bouncing to a minimum.

» **Hydration pack:** While packs made specifically for running are lightweight, comfortable, and allow you to carry a boatload of water and other items, you don't need to carry one unless you're running for hours or on a major mountain or desert adventure. Once you get into longer trail runs, pick up the nifty, informative little book called *Trailhead: The Dirt on All Things Trail Running* to learn about small and lightweight packs suitable for longer trail runs.

REFLECTIVE GEAR

Wearing clothes with reflective paneling, neon colors, or flashing lights increases your safety at all times of day but can be crucial at dawn and dusk (not just after dark or predawn). All sorts of accessories exist, from pullover vests to clip-on lights, blinking bracelets to details on clothing, to fully reflective apparel.

LIGHTS

If you do plan to run in the dark, go a step further than reflectors and arm yourself with a good light—be it a headlamp, handheld light, or wearable contraption with waist- or chest-mounted lights. Brightness is measured by lumens. Other variable factors include weight, comfort, minimal bounce, rechargeable versus battery-powered, and if the light is waterproof or not.

SUNBLOCK

Since you'll be spending more time in the great outdoors, now that you're becoming a runner, you'll want a good sunblock that won't grease up and slide down your sweaty body. Sport formulas generally fight that grossness.

Sucky thought zapped by this chapter:

"I don't have all the stuff."

"I don't know
who to go with."

FIND YOUR MATCH

Remember the "Know Thyself" quiz you took on page xii? You answered *yes* or *no* to questions about being an introvert, an animal lover, being supercompetitive or not. Let's dig deeper into what attracts you to potential running partners to help you find the perfect match.

"For some people who may be drawn to community, joining a running club or finding a group will work great," says sports psychologist Dr. Justin Ross, founder of Denver's MindBodyHealth psychology and counseling center. "For others, really having that alone time, that solitude, getting into nature on a solo run will work best in helping to find that best path forward to starting the running chapter of your life."

KEY NO. 5 TO MAKING RUNNING NOT SUCK: FIND YOUR MATCH

Finding the right partner or partners, male or female, two-legged or four-legged—or knowing you'd rather go it alone—can make a big difference in your running experience and motivation.

RUNNING CLUB OR GROUP

Maybe you played team sports as a kid and loved camaraderie within athletics. Or maybe being held accountable—by having set meet-up times and always having someone to run with—sounds like just the thing you need to kick off your running. Or maybe a friendly group of people just sounds like an appealing scenario for whatever reason.

Running clubs and groups come in all types, sizes, and most importantly, paces.

GROUPS AND PARTNERS MAKE YOU BETTER

You've heard it before: exercising in groups, or with one partner, is highly motivating. Not only does the group or partner make you accountable—you can't really bail on meeting your running partner at 6:00 a.m. unless you want to lose a friend—but being surrounded by others doing the same activity as you makes you better at that activity.

The *Journal of Social Sciences* published a study in 2010 stating, "Social comparison theory predicts exercise outcome such that participants gravitate toward the behavior (high fit or low fit) of those around them."

In other words, choose a group or partner that's slightly better/faster/fitter than you, and reap the benefits. Even if you don't, know that a group or partner environment naturally makes you push yourself.

WHAT TO EXPECT FROM A CLUB OR GROUP

It's possible to find or put together a running group, a handful of people you're compatible running with and can meet up with occasionally. But a cohesive group like that can take a while to assemble.

Running clubs differ from running groups in that they're easier to find already established—there are thousands of running clubs across the United States—and they're more formally organized and structured (though the runs themselves can be casual—running with a club doesn't necessarily mean you're signing up for a super-fast pace). As you settle into a groove with other members, you might even find a handful of people whose pace and running preferences match yours whom you can run with outside of the organized club runs.

Running clubs meet anywhere between one and seven days a week for organized group runs. These runs can vary from casual meet-ups to track workouts to trail runs to longer runs that are likely on weekends.

Running clubs sometimes also meet for social events outside of runs, like post-run beers or meals, volunteering at local races, or entering and traveling to races together. They can be social, serious, or seriously social.

Know that most running clubs charge dues. The fees go toward the coaching you'll receive when joining the club, as many clubs pick races to train for and offer training plans as well as group runs. Some clubs offer other benefits, like stretching and strength-training sessions. Dues also go toward club social events and often include discounted race entries, discounts from local retailers who sponsor the club, and more.

HASH HOUSE HARRIERS

Running clubs vary on how much emphasis they put on the social/fun/drinking aspect of their activities versus the seriousness of the running. The decades-old, worldwide Hash House Harriers go by the tagline of being a "drinking club with a running problem" and pride themselves on their partying. Before every group run, the Hash House Harriers send a "hare" out to set the course for that day's run. The hare sprinkles flour on the ground for clues, and the harriers take off on the course trying to chase down the hare. HHH runs end with drinking, the telling of dirty jokes (an indoctrination for new members), and other fun-spirited traditions.

HOW TO FIND A RUNNING CLUB

If a running club of any sort sounds intriguing, here's how to find one near you:

1. Either ask at your local running specialty store, if you have one, or do a web search for "Running clubs in [*your town goes here*]." Or check the national site for Road Runners Club of America (rrca.org).

2. Vet the information you track down via word-of-mouth or on the internet by reading vital information, such as how much the dues are and if you can afford them;[1] how many group runs are available to members during the week and if the meeting days and times work for your schedule; if the club is open to beginners and if a range of paces partake in group runs (this is something you can ask more about via email or a phone call if it's not on the club website); if the club's vibe through its wording on the website sounds like it'd be a good fit for you and your personality. If all that jibes with you and your goals, then proceed to step 3. If not, research the other clubs that show up in your web search in your area.

3. Show up for a group run. Clubs usually allow newcomers to check out at least one group run for free. Ask the club organizer (info found on club's website) which of the club's organized runs would be best for you to drop in to, and show up to participate. Know that no decent club drops anyone on a group run; there's always someone waiting at road, trail, or path junctions to make sure no runner is left behind. Also know that *all* paces are usually welcome at club runs, unless you accidentally join a professional running club.

4. If you enjoyed yourself on the group run, join the club!

---

1 Club dues may seem expensive, but if you compare them to a gym membership, an online dating service, and/or a personal trainer, they're a bargain . . . and it's possible you'll get all three out of the club experience.

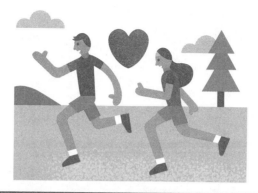

LOVE CONNECTION

Joining a group run might actually turn into a love connection. Spending a few miles running together on a road or trail in a nonthreatening, non-pressured environment can build great friendships. And sometimes much more.

WHAT TO WEAR TO A GROUP RUN

Not that you should overthink—or stress about—what to wear to a group run, but there are some things to consider . . . like the fact that you could be running up a steep trail in front of another runner, with your bum nearly at their eye level. In said situation, you don't really want to be wearing tights that have gotten too thin or shorts without a liner paired with underwear that doesn't securely hold your junk. And then there's the group stretching.

Wear whatever makes you the most comfortable and confident in a group situation. (Women, here's another argument for buying supportive sports bras.) And since you'll more than likely be driving or taking public transportation to the group run, you'll need a pocket for your keys, phone (if you want to carry one), and/or money/credit card. If you own running apparel that has a zippered pocket, wear it, or bring a small accessory that will hold your keys and/or other important items.[2]

---

2   See Chapter 4 for more on these options.

NO BOYS ALLOWED

Women's-only running clubs are a great asset to any level of female runner," says Dimity McDowell Davis, co-founder of Another Mother Runner and co-author of *Run Like a Mother*. "The runner who is just starting out discovers community (and motivation); the runner who is ready to push herself can find friend who is just a stitch faster than her; and veteran runners can share their experience and helpful tips (where, exactly, does one need body glide during a marathon?). Because clubs typically have all paces represented, everybody can find her pace in the pack—and enjoy the post-run chatter and coffee."

RUNNING PARTNER

If *one* platonic running partner to whom you're perfectly suited sounds appealing to you (maybe you're an introvert who enjoys one-on-one conversation, or groups just aren't your thing), then it's time for you to hunt for your match or matches.

> **BEGINNING RUNNER SEEKING LIKE-MINDED BEGINNING RUNNER. Must like piña coladas and getting caught in the rain.**

HOW TO FIND THE IDEAL RUNNING PARTNER

Finding the ideal running partner has some similarities to finding a life partner. Maybe you get a good partner vibe from someone in your running club; another participant at a race (if you do a race; see Chapter 10); or someone you see often or have seen on a running route you like. Or maybe you don't find your partner while you're actually running, but you discover that someone in your exercise class, office, school, or dorm is also interested in starting a non-sucky running routine and you think you might be able to bear (and maybe even enjoy!) logging some miles with them.

How can you find the right person? Take them out for a test spin, and ask yourself the following questions: Are we running at or around the same pace? Talking or not talking a similar amount? And when we are talking, do I like this person? Do they burp or fart (too much) while running? Do they generally annoy me? Do we have similar running goals and preferences (training for a race, or running for fitness or fun? trail runs or neighborhood loops? long or short runs?)?

TROUBLESHOOTING RUNNING PARTNER PROBLEMS

You may think you have the perfect running partner, and maybe you do. But like any relationship, problems can arise. Here's how to navigate them:

WHAT TO DO IF YOUR PARTNER IS RUNNING TOO FAST:

» **Quick fix:** Ask them an open-ended question like, "Are you religious?" or "Who was your first love?" while running, and they'll inevitably slow down while using their breath to talk.

» **Long term:** Have a heart-to-heart with them about paces and expectations. Schedule runs with them when you feel like a good ass-kicking or if you're mainly running with a partner for the accountability factor, and meet them at a designated time and place but let them know you're going to run at your own pace and that they can go ahead. Or meet them partway through their longer run (the later part), and run a shorter portion with them.

WHAT TO DO IF YOUR PARTNER IS RUNNING TOO SLOWLY:

» **Quick fix:** Slow your own pace, and get over it. It's OK to run slower than you intended once in a while.

» **Long term:** If they're insistent on partnering up day in and day out, have a heart-to-heart with them. Schedule runs with them when you need a recovery run, and don't feel badly about finding another partner or group (or go it alone) on days when you want to push your pace. You won't be satisfied with a run if, at the end, you know you didn't push yourself and you were looking to on that particular day. (But you'll survive if that does happen.)

WHAT TO DO IF YOUR PARTNER WON'T SHUT UP:

» **Quick fix:** Tell them that you're really going to focus on the running for a little while, or blurt out something shocking, like "I'm considering cannibalism!"

» **Long term:** If they don't get the hint, consider a new partner . . . like a dog.

WHAT TO TELL YOUR RUNNING PARTNER IF YOU'RE NOT IN THE MOOD/WOULD RATHER RUN ALONE THAT DAY:

» **Quick fix:** Explain that you already have plans to run with someone else and need to catch up one-on-one with that person (if this is true). Explain that you're getting more into mindful running and need to run solo for a while. Be honest and tell them you look forward to running with them the next time.

» **Long term:** If this becomes a regular feeling you have on the day you're slated to run with said partner, it's time to break up.

WHAT TO DO IF YOU WANT TO BREAK UP WITH YOUR RUNNING PARTNER:

» **Quick fix:** None (sorry); explain that you want to run alone for whatever reason; explain that maybe you're just not compatible as running partners.

» **Long term:** Don't do it over a text message; rather, have a heart-to-heart. Explain you want to run alone or that you aren't sure you're compatible partners for whatever reason (pace, time or location preferences, etc.). There's no need for a personal attack—stress personal running factors and preferences, and they should understand.

KEYS TO A HEALTHY RELATIONSHIP (WITH YOUR PLATONIC RUNNING PARTNER)

Treat your running partner relationship with care, as you would any other relationship in your life, to make sure it lasts.

- **MAKE SURE BOTH OF YOUR NEEDS ARE MET.** If your or your partner's running goals or nonnegotiables aren't being met (runs are way too fast or slow; you're meeting more or less frequently than you'd like; you or they talk too much or not enough; they're always late or bail last minute), they (or you) may be tempted to find another running partner. Be honest and up front about your preferences, ability, and goals when looking for a running partner, and maintain an open dialogue so that they know they can tell you if something's not working for them.

- **HAVE MUTUAL RESPECT.** Avoid talking down to your partner—there's a difference between friendly encouragement and condescending attempts to motivate. Respect their pace on any given day. And show up at the time you say you're going to meet them. Being on time is key in respecting a running partner.

- **COMPROMISE.** If your partner has different ideas from you about what you're doing that day, you may need to compromise. For instance, if you show up thinking you're running five miles together and they want to run one mile and go get a Slurpee at 7-Eleven, you may have to find a happy medium.

- **PRACTICE OPEN COMMUNICATION.** If the above scenario happens more than once, you two clearly aren't communicating well on expectations and needs. Time to have a talk (see "Troubleshooting Running Partner Problems").

- **TRUST EACH OTHER.** Like any relationship, trust is key. Running partners share personal stories on runs; there's something safe about being on a run with someone that makes the bond between two runners strong. But trust is imperative. Secrets shared on runs should be held sacred.

RUNNING WITH YOUR BAE

Some couples run together every day. Some couples break up after trying to run together once.

The same rules apply with a significant other running partner as with a platonic running partner, though, since more is at stake, there are more rules. Add to the previous tips the following:

» **Use conflict resolution.** Romantic couples tend to have more conflict than platonic couples. (More passion! More heated discussions! More fully loaded conversations! More grudges!) If you want to stay a couple, you can't very well just ditch them as a running partner with no explanation, so be sure to practice the first five rules of a healthy running relationship and adjust as necessary. Still not working? Save your relationship. Don't run together.

RUNNING WITH A DOG

If you're saying, " Awwww!" to yourself right now at the thought of a run with Fido, consider running with your—or a—dog. Maybe you own a dog capable of running, you're interested in getting a dog who can run, or you can borrow a friend's pup every once in a while.

Studies have long shown that owners of dogs take more steps per day than non-dog owners. (Gotta walk that dog!) Get yourself a pooch that needs to run or else they tear apart your furniture or act out in other ways, and you're bound to head out for runs and long walks more than not. Some dogs start wagging their tails or jumping up and down excitedly at the sight of your running shoes. Others learn to skillfully manipulate you with their puppy dog eyes when they're longing for a run.

Dogs can be ideal running partners. They go wherever and whenever you want, and not only do they not complain, they're eager and excited every time. In fact, having a dog can be highly motivating, as your dog needs exercise and depends on you to give him or her said exercise.

DOG BREEDS WELL-SUITED FOR RUNNING

There's a whole pack of dog breeds that are good runners, pets, and running pets. Here's a list to get you started, but be sure to research more to find the ideal partner for you.[3]

DOG BREED BEST FOR RUNNERS WHO:

Like to be licked	golden and Labrador retrievers
Like short-haired, big dogs	vizsla
Like short-haired, big dogs	Weimaraner
Like a dog who looks tough (half the time)	Rhodesian ridgeback
Like to be herded	border collie
Like to be herded	Australian shepherd
Like a dog who looks tough	German shepherd
Like insane small dogs	Jack Russell terrier
Have a Disney/firefighter fixation	dalmatian
Live in cold climes	Alaskan malamute
Live in cold climes	Siberian husky
Like short-haired, medium-sized dogs who can retrieve	German shorthaired pointer
Like sprinting, or chasing after their sprinting dog	greyhound
Like long-haired, medium-sized dogs (and don't live in tick country)	English setter
Like Snoopy	beagle
Like watching their dog chase squirrels	fox terrier
Like the idea of a dog carrying brandy	greater Swiss mountain dog
Like running near creeks and lakes	Portuguese water dog
Like saying, "Catahoula!"	Catahoula leopard dog
Like telling everyone how smart their dog is	standard poodle
Like scrappy, loveable conglomerates	mutt

3   There are more breeds than these twenty that are good for running partners.

HOW TO RUN WITH A DOG

Generally speaking, dogs should be roughly a year and a half to two years old before starting a running routine so their growth plates are closed enough to make it safe for them to run without hurting their joints. Every dog is different, however, so check with your veterinarian about how old your dog should be before you take him or her running. And if your dog is older and has slowed down in their golden years, let them set the pace and don't push them.

Keep in mind that your dog should ease into running, just as you should, so don't expect either of you to run for a big chunk of time right off the bat. Easing into running by running and walking will be best for both your health and your dog's.

BEST TYPES OF RUNS FOR DOGS

"Do your knees ache after running on a concrete sidewalk? Chances are, your dog feels the same way," says Dr. Sarah Wooten, veterinarian and cocreator of Vets Against Insanity: The Slightly Scandalous Card Game for Veterinary Professionals. "Hard surfaces, like concrete and asphalt, have the same kind of jarring impact on dog and human joints, so it is better to choose softer surfaces, like dirt or gravel trails, for runs with your dog. If all you have access to is a concrete jungle, then alternate running with brisk walking to minimize the pounding on your dog's joints."

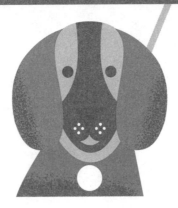

DOG-FRIENDLY RUNS: A QUIZ

How well did you pay attention to the previous advice?

1. My dog wants to train for a road marathon.

agree   disagree

2. My dog doesn't want to get dirty.

agree   disagree

3. My dog has too much pride to take walk breaks.

agree   disagree

4. My dog should buck up and run through pain on concrete road runs.

agree   disagree

5. My dog and I have absolutely nothing in common in relation to this topic.

agree   disagree

If you answered *agree* to all (or any) of the above questions, please reread the quote by veterinarian Sarah Wooten, above. Also, please reassess your own common sense.

WHAT TO TAKE WITH YOU ON A DOG RUN

First and foremost, never, ever, ever leave the house without a poop bag. That said, never leave your dog's poop where they decide to do their thing. Use the bag you brought and bag that shit up, carry it with you (yes, carry it with you) to the nearest trash can, and dispose of it properly. Nothing says "f*** you, neighbor," like letting your dog leave a deuce on their lawn. Even if you don't like your neighbor, don't do it.

Secondly, you need a leash. Running-specific dog leashes do exIst, some with contraptions that attach around your waist for hands-free running. Only use this kind of leash if your dog isn't obsessed with trying to chase and kill squirrels, chipmunks, rabbits, and butterflies, lest they take off after some would-be prey with you in tow. Regular leashes also work, if you don't mind holding one in hand.

Consider carrying extra water for your dog if you're going on a longer run or run/walk, especially in warm weather. Some dogs will drink if you squirt a water bottle near their mouths. Others prefer if you pour water into your hand and let them drink from your cupped palm. With others, you'll need to wait until you get back to your car or house. (Consider keeping extra water and a dog bowl—collapsible dog bowls are handy—in your car for this purpose.) And/or, run by water sources.

DOG LEASH LAWS

Some trails allow dogs off leash while others do not. And some trails allow only certain dogs off leash: dogs whose owners have gone through the process of getting a voice-control tag (worn by the dog) that indicates the dog responds to voice commands. Check leash laws in your area before letting your dog off leash.

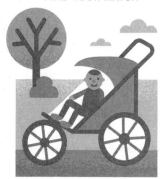

RUNNING WITH KIDS

Have young kids who like riding in the stroller (and/or need a nap)? Or older kids who could use a little energy burn-off? Maybe you never considered running with your kid or kids, but considering you're just starting out, now's the perfect time for this family bonding experience.

WIN-WIN FOR PARENTS AND KIDS

"As new parents, or parents of older kids, saying 'yes' to the needs of your kids and your family is easy, but saying 'no' to your own health will eventually come back and harm you," says sports psychologist Dr. Justin Ross. "Making time for yourself to exercise, to run, improves health, helps manage stress better, and gives parents an identity, a purpose, a sense of self they wouldn't get in just caring for the kids."

"And taking young kids out for runs in the stroller sets this pattern of living a healthy, active lifestyle. It's something they do, look forward to doing, and get excited about. And you're modeling to them this healthy way forward."

KIDS WHO FIT IN STROLLERS

Parents of young kids! The single best thing you can do for yourself, aside from getting some sleep, is to get your hands on a jogging stroller. Why?

Jogging stroller = Freedom

Little ones often fall asleep from the motion of being in a stroller. If they don't, they're still getting fresh air and outdoor stimulation, all while you get some exercise. Having a jogging stroller means you don't have to wait (or pay) for a babysitter to show up to get your exercise.

WHAT MAKES A STROLLER A JOGGING STROLLER?

Also called a *baby jogger* or a *running stroller*, these types of baby-wheeling devices have one wheel up front that locks into a straight position for safety while running (and unlocks for navigating grocery store aisles and the like) and two larger wheels in the back. All wheels are made of rubber, like bike tires, and filled with air. Other features include shock absorbers, hand brakes, parking brakes, storage pockets, and optional accessories like sippy cup holders.

WHAT TO BRING WITH YOU

If you're a parent to a baby or toddler, you already know never to leave the house without a whole slew of items. But here's a checklist for what to bring on a run with a baby in a jogger:

- ☐ Diapers and wipes
- ☐ Trash bag for storing dirty diapers
- ☐ Sippy cup/bottle and snacks for baby
- ☐ Blanket for baby
- ☐ Other items to bundle up/shield baby from sun
- ☐ Water/snacks for you

And since jogging strollers have such great storage pockets, you can bring with you whatever you want on your run, like extra layers, your phone, even a book to read (or work you can do) if your baby does fall asleep and you could use some quiet time after—or even during—your run.

EASING BACK INTO RUNNING FOR NEW MOMS

Some moms can't wait to get back to running after finally getting that baby out of their bodies. Since you thought running sucked before starting this book, you may or may not feel that way—maybe the thought of running with your baby is more motivating to you than running solo for whatever reason. Regardless, know that you need to be patient. Giving birth to another human takes a toll on all sorts of body parts, all of which need to recover before you start taxing them with running. Be sure to follow your doctor's guidance on when you can get back into running (usually six to eight weeks postdelivery) and how slowly you should ease into the practice (a run/walk routine is likely a good start to give your body a chance to adjust). This will vary person to person and be different for those who were avid runners before giving birth versus those who haven't run in years—so don't compare yourself to that new-mom friend of yours who's training for a marathon a month after giving birth to twins. Every body is different; be kind to yours.

EASING BACK INTO RUNNING FOR NEW DADS

Dads, just because you didn't birth the baby doesn't mean your body has gotten away scot-free (though refrain from complaining about that to your partner). Both parents need to take heed of all kinds of funky pains brought on by caring for babies: holding a baby on one hip can throw your body out of overall alignment; hunching over while holding baby in your arms and making *goo-goo, gaa-gaa* noises gives you rounded shoulders and a sore neck; a lack of sleep messes with your overall system.

You, as well as your baby's mama, need to *ease* into—or back into—running with care.

KIDS WHO DON'T FIT IN STROLLERS

While the American Academy of Pediatrics warns against kids running marathons, doctors advise that short distances, done safely and supervised, can be great for older middle school–aged kids and up. And since you're easing into running yourself, now's the perfect time to ease your kid into it, too. Talk to your family and see if anyone's interested in joining you on runs.

Running together, either in an organized race like a 5K or in an unorganized setting, can be a great bonding experience for you and your child. There's something about not facing each other—the same phenomenon that happens when parents drive their kids around—that allows both parties to open up and discuss things they wouldn't otherwise.

Many running races include kid-specific events, which can be a fun motivator to get your child running. Or your child could do the race you've chosen to do with you, like a 5K. (See Chapter 10 for more on racing.) Kids tend to love races because of their festive environment, free goodies, race T-shirts, and medals.

NEW-PARENT SURVIVAL EXERCISES

Try these exercises to combat common new-parent aches:

FOAM ROLLER CHEST OPENER

1. Lie on a foam roller so it runs lengthwise along your spine and supports you from your tailbone to your head.
2. Extend your arms as if you're doing a snow angel. Then, pretend to do a snow angel, moving your arms up overhead and down by your side, stopping and breathing for extra seconds in any positions that feel extra tight.

SHOULDER BLADE STRENGTHENER

1. Stand with your heels and back against a wall and with your arms bent to 90 degrees and pressed flat against the wall.
2. From 90 degrees, straighten and raise your arms up overhead.

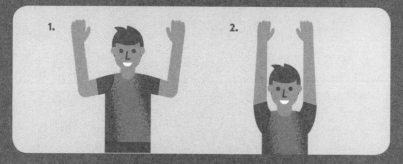

3. Return arms to starting position. Repeat ten to fifteen times, and do three sets.

HIP SWAP

A few times a day, carry that baby on the opposite hip. This will help alleviate the out-of-whack-ness you've likely gotten in your hips/pelvis from carrying baby on one hip every day. The goal is to stay/get symmetrical, not to create a shelf (one protruding hip) on one side of your body.

SLEEP

Get more of it. (Best of luck.)

RUNNING SOLO

If you answered *yes* to the question "Are you an introvert?" on page xii, solo runs are probably most appealing to you. But even if you're an extrovert and spend most of your time running with others, running alone once in a while can be a great way to have some quiet time alone (underrated!) and clear your mind.

PROS AND CONS TO RUNNING ALONE

PROS	CONS
• Time to yourself	• Can be lonely
• Time to think or not think	• Can allow you to think too much
• No breath wasted from talking	• Might miss talking to a friend/partner
• Pay attention to running form, or practice mindfulness (or mindlessness; see page 6)	• Become bored out of your mind from paying attention to form or from practicing mindfulness
• Go at your own pace	
• Go whenever works for you (without depending on or catering to someone else)	• Rock out so hard practicing mindlessness that you get lost or wander into traffic
• Go for however long you want	• Might be less likely to push yourself to run faster or longer
• Fart, burp, or blow snot rockets with wild abandon	• Easy to blow off a run
	• Must be more safety-aware than if you were with someone

SAFETY TIPS FOR SOLO RUNNERS

Since there is safety in numbers, you need to be more aware of your surroundings in both urban and natural settings when you're running solo than when you're with a partner or group.

If you head out for a run alone, take the following safety precautions:

- **Carry a phone.** Is it bulky? Yes. But it's important to have a way to call for help if you get injured or find yourself in some kind of danger. See page 77 for how to carry one comfortably.

- **Don't wear headphones.** In an urban area, you want to be able to hear footsteps or voices. In a natural area, you want to hear footsteps of animals—human or wild—rustling brush, and the like. If you can't run without music, wear one earbud instead of both or turn your volume down.

- **Make eye contact** with people you pass by, and say hello. This lets them know you see them (which can deter predators) and helps them remember seeing you, should you go missing for any reason.

- **Carry money or a credit card** in case you get too far from your starting point or are unexpectedly tired and need to take public transportation or a cab to get back safely—or in case you want to buy yourself a coffee or cold drink on your way back home. (Or you can access Uber or Lyft with your phone.)

- **Consider carrying self-protection.** Some solo runners feel safer when they carry a whistle or pepper spray or have an emergency safety SOS feature on their phone or smartwatch at the ready.

HOW TO MOTIVATE YOURSELF ON A SOLO RUN

Sometimes, being someone who likes to run alone can make it too easy to *not* go running at all. Or, if you make it out the door, you might be tempted to turn around and call it quits, since no one's watching or depending on you to keep going (besides you). To ward off the temptation of quitting when solo, set mini goals for yourself during the run. "Get to that stoplight without walking!" "Stay out thirty minutes today, even if I walk half the time!" (See Chapter 6 for run/walk plans along these lines.) And then reward yourself for completing your goal. Beer! Hot bath! *Real Housewives* binge!

MIX IT UP

While introverts will thrive on solo runs and extroverts will thrive in company, it's healthy for both types to mix things up once in a while. Introverts can benefit—socially and in their running—from running in groups or with one partner on occasion. If you fall into the introverted group, schedule in some time to run with humans of some sort. Dogs are great, but runs with them don't count as social runs. Running with a human occasionally can also help gauge your fitness, so you can go back to running without any annoying humans and keep improving on your own.

Extroverts can also benefit from running alone. Being extroverted can be exhausting, and making the time you spend running a reprieve from all that socializing you normally do can help you recharge and return to your otherwise social world with more energy than ever. If you're an extrovert, schedule in some time to run solo once in a while. And for you, running with a dog counts as running alone, unless you have a talking dog. Also consider either not touching your phone on your run or leaving it at home. Answering calls or posting to social media mid-run count as being social. Instead, savor the quiet time to yourself.

Sucky thought zapped by this chapter:

"I don't want to run alone (or do I?)."

WAYPOINT

Now that you've figured out the best way for you, and specifically you, to approach running, how do you feel about it?

Does it seem slightly less sucky?

It's okay if you're not jumping for joy at the mention of the word *running*. It's a journey.

Jot down your thoughts on the facing page, or doodle a picture and give yourself a Rorschach test to interpret your feelings. Take a second to think about how your attitude toward running might have changed over the last five chapters. Or don't write anything and tear that page out and use it for a grocery list.

How I feel about running *now*:

_____

_____

_____

_____

_____

_____

_____

_____

_____

_____

_____

_____

_____

_____

_____

_____

_____

_____

"I can't run more than ten minutes straight."

START WHERE YOU ARE

Honestly, if you spontaneously decide one day to go out and try to run a certain number of minutes or miles straight—whether you're coming from the couch or from spin class—it *is* going to suck. Everything will hurt, and you'll likely hate the experience.

Training plans exist (online, in books, via apps, from coaches in person) to help runners at any level improve safely, without injuring themselves, and successfully . . . whether their goal is to eventually complete a certain distance, clock a certain time, improve in another sport, or simply get fitter. But diving into a generic training plan without a little personalization can make running, well, suck.

So where to begin? Since the first step in achieving any of the above goals is to learn to actually stomach—and eventually maybe even love—running, do this: start where you are. That means both physically (see categories on page 110) and in terms of your personality—what sounds fun to you—and gets you even remotely excited about running.

KEY NO. 6 TO MAKING RUNNING NOT SUCK: START WHERE YOU ARE

Forget about thinking you "should" be able to run a certain amount of time or miles or at a certain pace. Self-assess where you are, what type of runs might actually appeal to you, and ease into running slowly (alternating running and walking, if that's where you are) for a successful and enjoyable buildup.

SO, WHERE ARE YOU?

Someone who's never run before and isn't generally very active in their daily life will have a different starting point from someone who, say, plays rugby twice a week but hates going running, or someone who (begrudgingly) runs regularly. For that reason, here are four categories that should help you home in on a starting point for becoming a runner—a runner who doesn't hate every step.

YOU ARE:

» **HERE: Never Ever, Like Ever** ●○○○

You've never been a runner. You never played sports of any sort—or if you did, it was years and years (and years) ago. You're starting from what feels like square one.

» **HERE: Returning Athlete** ●●○○

You did sports of some sort in the not-too-distant past. You still have some muscle memory—and even some muscle—but you never really considered yourself a runner. Running was something you did back in the day to stay in shape for your sport, but you didn't and don't seek it out. Maybe you're starting from square two.

» **HERE: Non-Running Current Athlete** ●●●○

You do sports[1] or work out in some form now, so your body is used to being pushed, but you don't currently run consecutive steps beyond chasing after a tennis ball or sprinting to get to the elliptical before the person who hogs it. Square three!

» **HERE: Intermittent Runner (Who Hates It)** ●●●●

You run occasionally, whether it's during a gym workout or on your own. You hate it, so you don't do it that often and curse every step. You have all the squares, but

---

1   Soccer, Ultimate Frisbee players, and other run-heavy sports players can be considered intermittent runners—see next level.

maybe you've been trying fit a square peg into a round hole. You have friends or read about people who seem to actually enjoy and look forward to running, and you crave a new mind-set to help you learn to love it.

The running plans in this book are specifically created for all four types of people who think running sucks and don't want to start a running plan. Something got you to read this far. Trust that feeling. Read on. You'll find a unique approach that works for unique you.

CAVEATS

Only want to run two days a week? No problem! Do your other stuff (go on a walk, go to the gym, play a shit-ton of video games if that's your thing) in between your two running days. Want to lace up a fourth day? Awesome. Just make sure you don't do two days back-to-back while you're starting out.

RUNNING IS DIFFERENT

Even if you do a ton of other aerobic sports—mountain biking, road cycling, swimming, Nordic skiing, CrossFit, and so on— you'll still need to ease into running. Specific muscles and joints are used in running that aren't in other sports, and due to the repetitive nature of running, they're used a lot. That's why the running plans to follow integrate walk breaks and build up slowly so that you gradually train those running-specific muscles and joints and ward off injury. And, so that you might actually focus on the good parts of running and keep with it.

CHECK-INS

A lot of people make the mistake of starting a specific training plan and forcing themselves to stick to it verbatim, no matter how they're feeling physically or mentally. They end up resenting the plan . . . and resenting running in general.

To avoid such resentment, it's important to check in with yourself throughout whichever approach/plan you choose to pursue and adjust as necessary to help you keep the love flowing.

"If you feel like going harder, go harder," says Scott Fliegelman, who founded Boulder, Colorado–based FastForward Sports and acted as head coach for ten years, helping thousands of athletes find joy in running. "If you feel like going easier, do. Listening to yourself is important. And whatever pace you run, you're a runner."

EMBRACE THE RUN/WALK

Since inventing a method he coined "Run-Walk-Run" in 1974, coach Jeff Galloway has transformed thousands of people who never thought they could run into capable—even marathon-finishing—athletes. His training plans lay out alternating running with walking in increments as short as fifteen seconds. "Run-Walk-Run puts you in control over how you feel during and after a run," he explains.

Galloway says alternating running and walking by a prescribed amount of time, as opposed to a distance, keeps beginners from running too far when they're starting out. But, he says, both can work. "The simplest form of the method is to take a walk break so early in the run that muscle fatigue is erased and stress on weak links goes away," he says. "If you don't feel good, reduce the running segments and increase the frequency of the walking. There never has to be suffering."

LEARN-TO-LOVE RUNNING PLANS

On the following pages, you'll find plans for each type of runner—Never Ever, Like Ever; Returning Athlete; Non-Running Current Athlete; and Intermittent Runner (Who Hates It)—based on different approaches to running that suit different personalities. Start your path to loving running with a method that best suits *you*, choosing an approach that goes by *time*, by *feel*, by *distances* on the track or elsewhere (i.e., telephone poles in your neighborhood, lifeguard towers on the beach), by *music* in your ears, or by a more *abstract approach based on time*.

And since each type of runner has a different starting point as far as current fitness is concerned, you'll have a different starting point within each plan.

All of these plans are based on putting on running shoes and heading out the door (which makes you a runner no matter how much you're walking, what speed you're traveling, or how frequently you're doing it) two to three times a week. Just don't do your run/walk days back-to-back to start. And all plans that follow are kept to thirty minutes long, because if you hate something, you probably don't really want to be doing it for more than thirty minutes, at least until about seven weeks in. Although, if you want to stay out longer, by all means, do! Just walk for longer instead of adding more running too soon.

DREAM COME TRUE

"I started having dreams in my midtwenties about being able to run and feeling really free, but I had asthma and never thought I could do it. A few years ago, a runner friend took me out, and we walked mostly but ran one minute at a time with walk breaks in between, just a few times at first. She taught me how to control my breath by breathing slowly, in through my nose and out through my mouth. The fact that the run portions were only one minute long also helped me control my breathing and kept my asthma in check.

"I ran a 5K nine weeks later and have run at least ten since then. I love that a run gives me an escape to clear my mind and some alone time, which I don't get very often as a working mom. I feel great."

—Alex Gilbert, 40, Firestone, Colorado

PACE SCHMACE, FORM SCHMORM

Do not worry about how fast or slow you might be running when you first start out. Running can mean picking up your feet slightly more than you would while walking. "A mistake some people make when alternating running and walking is running too fast and using walk breaks as a crutch to recover," says running coach, author, and nutritionist Matt Fitzgerald. "There is no harm in going out too easy, especially when you're starting out." (For advice on how to get faster, or if hard efforts sound fun to you, turn to page 203.)

Same goes for form. There are numerous books, coaches, and gurus of all sorts who preach how to run "properly," and there is a ton of merit in good form. But when you're just starting out, just run however feels most natural to you. Don't worry about high knees, landing on your midfoot, dancing lightly, or channeling your ancestors while they chased down their dinner. Just shuffle along however feels the most natural. You can work on form later.

LEARN TO LOVE RUNNING: BY TIME

» **Best if you:** Don't mind having your hand held a little; want a fairly fail-safe method to easing into running; are a rule-follower; don't mind frequently looking down at your wrist.

» **Needed:** A watch. (A digital chronograph watch is easiest to follow and can be preset to beep at you when it's time to run or walk.)

» **Where:** Outside on the road, a trail, the track, or inside on a treadmill. If you do it on a trail or on hilly terrain on the road, you'll need to adjust a bit based on feel: run for longer on a downhill, shorter on an uphill.

» **How:** Unless you have a photographic memory, either cut out the workout to take with you, or jot it down on something small like a business card and take that with you. Alternatively, you could try to memorize it, and/or you could take a picture of it with your phone to reference if you forget (and don't mind taking your phone with you). Some watches can be preset.

WEEK 1   ●○○○
NEVER-EVER: START HERE

- Lace up 2–3 times a week

- 2 minutes total of running, 4 × 30 seconds

» 0:00–10:00 walk

» 10:00–10:30 jog/pick up your feet slightly more than you would when walking

» 10:30–12:30 walk

» 12:30–13:00 jog/pick up your feet slightly more than you would when walking

» 13:00–15:00 walk

» 15:30–16:00 jog/pick up your feet slightly more than you would when walking

» 16:00–18:00 walk

» 18:00–18:30 jog/pick up your feet slightly more than you would when walking

» 18:30–30:00 walk

WEEK 2   ●○○○

- Lace up 2–3 times a week

- 3 minutes total of running, 4 × 45 seconds

» 0:00–10:00 walk

» 10:00–10:45 jog/pick up your feet slightly more than you would when walking

» 10:45–12:30 walk

» 12:30–13:15 jog/pick up your feet slightly more than you would when walking

» 13:15–15:00 walk

» 15:00–15:45 jog/pick up your feet slightly more than you would when walking

» 15:45–17:15 walk

» 17:15–18:00 jog/pick up your feet slightly more than you would when walking

» 18:00–30:00 walk

CHECK YO SELF: AN EVALUATION

After this week, how are you feeling?

☐ **Feisty?** Consider adding a little time to your run increments (skip ahead to a future week's plan); walking for longer at the end of your run increments; or going for a brisk walk on a day or two between runs.

☐ **Sluggish/Annoyed?** Consider running shorter or slower during your run increments, and repeat this week's plan before moving on to Week 3. Or consider going on a hike or bike ride in a pretty place (or in a dirty alley, if that's your thing) instead of one of your runs.

☐ **Fine?** Continue on to the next week.

WEEK 3 ●○○○
WEEK 1 ●●○○

RETURNING ATHLETE: START HERE. IT'S YOUR WEEK 1.

- Lace up 2–3 times a week

- 4 minutes of running, 4 × 1 minute

» 0:00–10:00 walk

» 10:00–11:00 jog/pick up your feet slightly more than you would when walking

» 11:00–13:00 walk

» 13:00–14:00 jog/pick up your feet slightly more than you would when walking

» 14:00–16:00 walk

» 16:00–17:00 jog/pick up your feet slightly more than you would when walking

» 17:00–19:00 walk

» 19:00–20:00 jog/pick up your feet slightly more than you would when walking

» 20:00–30:00 walk

WEEK 4 ●○○○
WEEK 2 ●●○○

- Lace up 2–3 times a week

- 6 minutes of running, 4 × 90 seconds

- The jump in running is 30 seconds instead of 15; you're ready for it. If you'd rather, throw in a terrain change, like a gradual uphill, and keep running increments at 1 minute when on hills, making them longer when on downhills.

» 0:00–10:00 walk

» 10:00–11:30 jog/pick up your feet slightly more than you would when walking

» 11:30–13:00 walk

» 13:00–14:30 jog/pick up your feet slightly more than you would when walking

» 14:30–16:00 walk

» 16:00–17:30 jog/pick up your feet slightly more than you would when walking

» 17:30–19:00 walk

» 19:00–20:30 jog/pick up your feet slightly more than you would when walking

» 20:30–30:00 walk

CHECK YO SELF: AN EVALUATION

After this week, how are you feeling?

☐ **Feisty?** Consider adding a little time to your run increments (skip ahead to a future week's plan), a little speed[2] to your run increments, or hills.[3] Or consider walking for longer at the end of your run increments, or go for a brisk walk on your days off from running.

☐ **Sluggish/Annoyed?** Consider running shorter (you could go back to a prior week's plan), or slower during your run increments or going on a hike or bike ride—maybe a harder one than in previous weeks—in a pretty place instead on one of your run days. Or do a fun workout or class at a gym. The point is to do something active that sounds fun.

☐ **Fine?** Continue on to the next week.

....

2 If you feel like running fast, do your run intervals (maybe slightly shorter) at a more intense pace, recovering for a little longer on your walking intervals. Do this only once a week, however, to help mitigate injury.
3 A hill does not mean a mountain. A hill is anything that is a slight incline; if you put a marble on it, it would roll backward, however slowly. You can achieve the effect of a hill by increasing the treadmill incline by a percentage, or running on a road or trail in your neighborhood that isn't flat or downhill. And then, of course, you can progress from there and go steeper as you get stronger.

WEEK 5 ●○○○
WEEK 3 ●●○○
WEEK 1 ●●●○

NON-RUNNING CURRENT ATHLETE: START HERE. IT'S YOUR WEEK 1.

- Lace up 2–3 times a week

- 10 minutes of running, 4 × 2:30

» 0:00–10:00 walk

» 10:00–12:30 jog/pick up your feet slightly more than you would when walking

» 12:30–13:30 walk

» 13:30–16:00 jog/pick up your feet slightly more than you would when walking

» 16:00–17:00 walk

» 17:00–19:30 jog/pick up your feet slightly more than you would when walking

» 19:30–21:30 walk[4]

» 21:30–24:00 jog/pick up your feet slightly more than you would when walking

» 23:00–30:00 (or longer, but not shorter) walk

WEEK 6 ●○○○
WEEK 4 ●●○○
WEEK 2 ●●●○

- Lace up 2–3 times a week

- 12 minutes of running, 4 × 3 minutes. Or throw in a terrain change like a gradual uphill, and keep running increments shorter when on hills, making them longer when on downhills. Or throw in a speed change, running harder during the run increments, and walking slower to recover.

» 0:00–8:00 walk

----

4 This walk increment is longer than the others because the run increments have gotten longer.

» 8:00–11:00 jog/run

» 11:00–12:00 walk

» 12:00–15:00 jog/run

» 15:00–16:00 walk

» 16:00–19:00 jog/run

» 19:00–21:00 walk[5]

» 21:00–24:00 jog/run

» 24:00–30:00 (or longer, but not shorter) walk

CHECK YO SELF: AN EVALUATION

After this week, how are you feeling?

☐ **Feisty?** Consider adding a little time to your run increments (skip ahead to a future week's plan), a little speed to your run increments, or hills. Or consider walking for longer at the end of your run increments or going for a brisk walk on your days off from running.

☐ **Sluggish/Annoyed?** Considering running shorter (go back to a prior week's plan) or slower during your run increments, or going on a hike or bike ride in a pretty place instead on one of your run days. Or take a day off altogether . . . especially if you're starting to have trouble sleeping, which could indicate you're doing too much right now.

☐ **Fine?** Continue on to the next week.

....

5   This walk increment is longer than the others because the run increments have gotten longer.

WEEK 7 ●○○○
WEEK 5 ●●○○
WEEK 3 ●●●○
WEEK 1 ●●●●

INTERMITTENT RUNNER WHO HATES IT: START HERE. IT'S YOUR WEEK 1.

- Lace up 2–3 times a week

- 18 minutes of running, 4 × 4 minutes, plus 1 × 2 minutes

» 0:00–5:00 walk

» 5:00–9:00 jog/run

» 9:00–9:30 walk

» 9:30–13:30 jog/run

» 13:30–14:00 walk

» 14:00–18:00 jog/run

» 18:00–18:30 walk

» 18:30–22:30 jog/run

» 22:30–23:00 walk

» 23:00–25:00 jog/run

» 25:00–30:00 (or longer, but not shorter) walk

WEEK 8 ●○○○
WEEK 6 ●●○○
WEEK 4 ●●●○
WEEK 2 ●●●●

- Lace up 2–3 times a week

- 23 minutes of running, 4 × 5 minutes, plus 1 × 3 minutes. Or throw in a terrain change like a gradual uphill, and keep running increments shorter when on hills, making them longer when on downhills. Or throw in a speed change, running harder during the run increments and walking slower to recover.

» 0:00–5:00 walk

» 5:00–10:00 jog/run

» 10:00–10:30 walk

» 10:30–15:30 jog/run

» 15:30–16:00 walk

» 16:00–21:00 jog/run

» 21:00–21:30 walk

» 21:30–26:30 jog/run

» 26:30–27:00 walk

» 27:00–30:00 jog/run

» 30:00–35:00 (or longer, but not shorter) walk

CHECK YO SELF: AN EVALUATION

After this week, how are you feeling?

☐ **Feisty?** Add a little time to your run increments (skip ahead to a future week's plan), a little speed to your run increments, or add hills. Or consider walking for longer at the end of your run increments, or go for a brisk walk on your days off from running.

☐ **Sluggish/Annoyed?** Considering running shorter (go back to a prior week's plan), or slower during your run increments, or going on a hike, bike ride, or pub crawl instead of one of your run days. Or take a nap.

☐ **Fine?** Continue on to the next week.

WEEK 9 ●○○○
WEEK 7 ●●○○
WEEK 5 ●●●○
WEEK 3 ●●●●

- Lace up 2–3 times a week

- 26 minutes of running, 3 × 7:30, 1 × 3:30

» 0:00–5:00 walk

» 5:00–12:30 jog/run

» 12:30–13:30 walk

» 13:30–21:00 jog/run

» 21:00–22:00 walk

» 22:00–29:30 jog/run

» 29:30–30:30 walk

» 30:30–34:00 jog/run

» 34:00–40:00 (or longer, but not shorter) walk

WEEK 10 ●○○○
WEEK 8 ●●○○
WEEK 6 ●●●○
WEEK 4 ●●●●

- Lace up 2–3 times a week

- 30 minutes of running, 3 × 10 minutes

» 0–5:00 walk

» 5:00–15:00 jog/run

» 15:00–16:00 walk

» 16:00–26:00 jog/run

» 26:00–27:00 walk

» 27:00–37:00 jog/run

» 37:00–42:00 (or longer, but not shorter) walk

ONWARD

- **Improve.** From here, increase the run segments by two minutes per segment.

- **Improve more.** From there, increase the run segments to 2 × 15 minutes.

- **Improve even more.** After your five-minute walking warm-up, run 20–25 minutes straight. Add minutes to that run time as you progress.

> NOTE: If you already run for 30+ minutes or a certain amount of time straight, but hate it, try a) short walking breaks; b) mixing up when and where; and c) adhering to other tips in this book regarding mindshift, gear, company, etc.

CROSS-TRAINING

Cross-training—activities besides running—are great in that they keep your body moving without stressing the muscles and joints used in running, allowing you to be active on "off" days from running, if you want to be.

Non-Running Current Athletes and Intermittent Runners (Who Hate It) likely already cross-train.

Cross-training activities include:

- cycling
- walking
- gardening
- rock climbing
- swimming
- weight lifting
- skiing/snowboarding
- hiking
- Nordic skiing
- rowing
- yoga
- Pilates
- ball sports
- elliptical machining
- dancing

Note: If you do an activity that uses your legs—like hiking, walking, skiing/snowboarding, cycling, rowing, using the elliptical, or playing ball sports—factor that into how much time you need to recover before another run, or take your next run easier than you would if you didn't use your legs the day before. Even though a cross-training activity may not use the same exact muscles, those activities take a toll. If you do an activity that's aerobic—like cycling, swimming, rowing, or Nordic skiing as your cross-training—factor that in to your needed rest for recovery as well. For instance, don't do a feisty, harder-interval run the day after a hard swim or bike ride.

LEARN TO LOVE RUNNING: ABSTRACTLY, BY TIME

» **Best if you:** Have a rebellious streak and want a looser approach to increasing running by time

» **Needed:** A watch

» **Where:** On a road, a trail, a treadmill, a track

» **How:**
1. Walk for roughly the first five minutes. If you feel like walking for six, go nuts.

2. Run until you don't effing feel like running anymore. Maybe this is 30 seconds, maybe it's a few minutes.

3. Walk again, dammit.

4. Run again, laughing in the face of structure. (Or just run.)

5. Repeat for the remainder of your run, aiming to run for a total of 2 or 3 minutes on your first time out. Break down those 2 or 3 minutes within a 30-minute outing however the hell you want. The other 27 or 28 minutes, walk.

6. Walk to cool down.
   - **Improve (Week 3ish):** Increase your total run time to 5 minutes.
   - **Improve more (Week 5ish):** Increase your total run time to 10 minutes. And walk more if you bloody feel like it.
   - **Improve even more (Week 7ish):** Increase your total run time to 15, 20, and eventually 30 minutes or more.

> **Tip:** Make sure you're entering this plan, and any other, from where you are physically and mentally as a runner. If you're an Intermittent Runner (Who Hates It), for instance, do the above by running, say, 20–30 minutes total, broken down however you want, for your first time out.

THINK LIKE A KID!

Think about how fun it was to run when you were a kid. If you can tap into that childlike feeling of running for fun—across a playground, in a kickball game, chasing after a kid you liked—you might just have the mind shift you need to really start enjoying yourself on the run.

LEARN TO LOVE RUNNING: BY FEEL

» **Best if you:** Don't love watches; need a break from technology; want to feel more in tune with your body

» **Needed:** An ability to listen to your body and mind

» **Where:** Anywhere

» **How:**

1. Start by walking.

2. When your body feels moderately warmed up (less creaky than when you started; usually about 5 to 10 minutes in), break into a jog.

3. Stop running and start walking when you still feel sorta okay, but when you notice a hitch in your stride or a light strain (more than usual) in your muscles or breath. *Do not* wait to walk until you can't breathe or talk.[6]

4. Start running again.

5. Repeat steps 3 and 4 three or four times.

....

6 The Talk Test: If you can no longer speak a full sentence, it's time to slow down and walk. Walk until you regain your breath and your muscles feel semi-ready. (Don't wait until you feel perfect, because you won't.)

6. Walk for a few minutes after your last run segment to cool down.
   - **Improve (Week 3ish):** Run for longer during each segment, but don't make jumps that are too big. Give yourself at least two to three runs with similar run-length segments before adding time.
   - **Improve more (Week 5ish):** Run for longer still during each segment. Again, do this gradually.
   - **Improve even more (Week 7ish):** You got it. Run for longer during each segment, still listening to your body.

> **Tip:** Choosing natural markers, as in "Run until that big tree," "Walk until the stop sign," can help motivate . . . but if your body tells you to stop before then, listen.

YOU WON'T ALWAYS FEEL SUCKY

"It takes time for the body to adapt to the demands of running," says Jenny Hadfield, running coach and coauthor of *Running for Mortals: A Commonsense Plan for Changing Your Life with Running.* "At first, it may seem really challenging. The more you ease into it, the easier it will be for your body to adapt and progress. You can expect to feel stronger within thirty days of regular training three times per week, with a training plan that progresses gradually from your current fitness."

LEARN TO LOVE RUNNING: WITH MUSIC

» **Best if you:** Need music to make your heart beat; don't like watches but want some structure on your runs; can't fathom getting out the door without music blasting in your ears

» **Needed:** Some way to play music into your ears and carry said music player comfortably (see page 77)

» **Where:** Anywhere

» **How:**

1. Walk for the duration of two songs (avoiding jam band epics).

2. Jog/run for the first verse of the next song.

3. Walk during the next verse and chorus of that song.

4. Jog/run for another verse, before walking until the end of the song.

5. Repeat the run/walk for four songs.

6. Walk home during the duration of two songs to cool down.
   - **Improve (Week 3ish):** Warm up by walking for two songs. Once you feel comfortable jog/running for the duration of a verse, increase the jog/run duration from one verse to two.
   - **Improve more (Week 5ish):** Warm up by walking for two songs. Jog/run for two verses and through the end of the chorus (while still walking for the rest of the song). Repeat for four songs.
   - **Improve even more (Week 7ish):** Warm up by walking for one or two songs. Jogging for an entire song, then walk a song, then jog/run for another entire song. Repeat for four or so songs.

Tip: Playing the same music/playlist will help you gauge your improvement.

Another tip: The cadence of a song can affect the speed with which your feet hit the ground, so choose songs accordingly. Look for a running playlist online or just choose songs that have an upbeat tempo. It's tough to crank out miles to "The Way You Look Tonight," unless you want to force yourself to run slower. Likewise, especially if you're first starting out, avoid superfast dance beats. You don't want the cadence of a song to make you feel badly about your stride or make you trip on yourself trying to keep up.

LEARN TO LOVE RUNNING: BY DISTANCE ON A TRACK

» **Best if you:** Are a visual thinker; feel more comfortable in controlled environments; are competitive

» **Needed:** A track

» **Where:** A track

» **How:**

1. Walk two laps.

2. Jog/shuffle the curve of the beginning of the third lap.

3. Walk the rest of the lap.

4. Jog/shuffle the curve of the beginning of the fourth lap.

5. Walk a cool down lap or two.

6. Walk two laps.

- **Improve (Week 3ish):** Walk two laps. Jog/shuffle the straightaway and half a curve, walking the rest of the lap. Repeat for four laps total. Walk two laps.
- **Improve more (Week 5ish):** Walk two laps. Jog/shuffle the straightaway and curve of the third lap (half a lap!), walking the rest of the lap. Repeat for four laps total. Walk two laps.
- **Improve even more (Week 7ish):** Walk two laps. Jog/shuffle a lap, walk a lap. Repeat for four laps (running two laps total). Walk two laps.

> **Tip:** If you get bored, try music in your ears.

> **Another tip:** While you're trying hard, take an inside lane. While you're not, move to an outside lane. Always look over your shoulder before switching lanes so you avoid collisions and annoyed track mates. For more on track etiquette, see page 188.

A NEED FOR SPEED

"I'm in the gym working out all the time, but I don't really like running on the road or on trails. It wasn't until I went to the track and ran hard that I realized I actually love running. I love going fast and pushing really hard and then lying on the ground feeling completely destroyed between intervals. I hadn't felt that before with running and realized I'd really missed going fast like I used to during tennis sprints and sprinting around the field when I used to play rugby."

—James Scheurer, 21, Boulder, Colorado

LEARN TO LOVE RUNNING: BY DISTANCE, NOT ON A TRACK

» **Best if you:** Are a visual thinker; don't want to go by time

» **Needed:** An ability to listen to your body (see "Learn to Love Running: By Feel"); a treadmill, if doing this on a treadmill; a GPS-enabled device (see Chapter 4), if doing this by device

» **Where:** On a road, a trail, a treadmill

» **How:**
1. Walk until your body feels less creaky than when you started.

2. Spot something ahead of you, but not too far ahead of you—a tree, a telephone pole, a stop sign. If you're on a treadmill or if going by distance measured by a device, choose a distance.

3. Jog/run to that thing/mileage.

4. Walk until another thing—a different tree, a different telephone pole, a yield sign. Or to the next mileage increment on your treadmill console or smartwatch.

5. Repeat, listening to your body. If the thing/increment you chose makes you go into overload—your muscles or lungs scream—walk sooner. Likewise, if you feel ready to run again before the first thing you chose, adjust said thing. Pick something closer/shorter.

6. Walk to cool down.
    - **Improve (Week 3ish):** Pick natural markers or distances on the treadmill or smartwatch that are farther than the first time you tried this.
    - **Improve more (Week 5ish):** Pick natural markers that are farther still and/or choose natural markers for your walking breaks that are closer together.
    - **Improve even more (Week 7ish):** Choose natural markers that are farther than you ever thought you could run at one time, only after you've built up to doing so.

> **Tip:** If you run the same route once a week, you'll be able to gauge your progress easily. That said, don't run the same route every time you head out. Your body wants to run varied routes, as does your mind.

PALM TREE TO PALM TREE

"I play volleyball every day and consider myself a good athlete, but the timed mile in PE was kind of challenging for me. Growing up, I never really liked running, but I wanted to get better. I started off running on the beach near my house. I set small goals like running to a palm tree twenty houses down, walking to catch my breath, and then running again, giving myself breaks to recharge. Before this, I never really enjoyed running, but giving myself breaks and being in a beautiful environment definitely helped."

—Alex Lougeay, 16, Encinitas, California

Sucky thought zapped by this chapter:

"I don't know how to start."

"It hurts."

COMMON PAINS IN THE ASS (AND OTHER BODY PARTS) AND HOW TO TREAT THEM

There's no denying the fact that running can hurt. While bettering your body and your mind, running also causes discomfort (sometimes, straight-up pain) . . . and the thought of this may have kept you from running in the past. It's important to know that some pains are *good* pains—and runners are known to become addicted to them. (In fact, those good pains—yes, even if they're uncomfortable—mean you're getting stronger.) Others are *not-so-good* pains—and those can both keep you from running (don't celebrate yet) and from general enjoyment of your day-to-day life. But even those not-so-good pains aren't always as bad as they seem.

Think of signs of discomfort—muscle soreness, heavy breathing—as signs of your body working harder, recovering, and getting into kick-ass shape. Some go so far as to say that getting out of their comfort zone by running and doing other exercise helps them to feel alive. And keep your eye on the prize: that amazing feeling you have when you're done with a run. (See Chapter 1.) Soon enough, you'll crave those feelings and realize they're important to improving as a runner.

But nasty, run-thwarting pain? That's your body's way of saying, "Pay attention. Slow down. Something's not quite right." Think of those severe pains as check-engine lights, warning you to pay closer attention to a particular body part before you do real damage. It's important to distinguish discomfort from pain.

DISCOMFORT/GOOD PAIN = YOU'RE WORKING HARD AND IMPROVING! YOU'RE CHALLENGING YOURSELF!

» **Muscle soreness:** You're getting stronger!

» **Elevated heart rate:** Look how well your heart works!

» **Burning lungs:** Look how well your lungs work!

These responses may take a while to kick in as a new runner, but they will. Just you wait.

NOT-SO-GOOD PAIN = CRANKY ACHE IN ONE SPECIFIC BODY PART (I.E., ONE KNEE) . . . OUCH!

» **Sharp pain** that comes on suddenly mid-run . . . ouch!

» **Dull ache** in a specific body part with every step . . . ouch!

» **All-over pain** from tripping on a run . . . ouch!

Generally speaking, discomfort/good pain doesn't injure you, while not-so-good pain can if you don't heed the warning it's trying to give you. And there are ways to mitigate common running pains and ailments, both by preventing them from happening in the first place and by treating them properly if they do.

KEY NO. 7 TO MAKING RUNNING NOT SUCK: KEEP YOUR PARTS WORKING

Running can hurt, but it can also let you know you're alive and well. Being able to tell the difference between discomfort and pain, and treating said pains properly, can keep you running like a well-oiled machine. Vroom.

YOUR BODY: AN OWNER'S MANUAL

Before starting any exercise plan, it is advised to be cleared by a doctor to protect yourself and the service life of your . . . life. The goal: keep the car/body running smoothly.

HOW LONG IT HURTS

Generally speaking, if pain comes on at the beginning of a run and then goes away during the run, it's something to notice and keep an eye on. If the pain persists or comes back in the twelve to twenty-four hours after a run, pay attention to that, too. If it's not gone after twenty-four hours, or lingers longer than twenty-four hours, consider seeing a practitioner of some sort. But don't freak out. Freaking out can make pain worse. (See page 153 for practitioners.)

A 2018 study published in the *Journal of Pain*, the official journal of the American Pain Society, found that stress can dramatically affect the body's ability to modulate and regulate pain. Researchers found there was a direct correlation between pain intensification and a decrease in pain inhibition capabilities due to psychological stress.

The takeaway: the less you can stress about a pain in your body, the better.

> **Don't forget:** Start slowly. The entire last chapter hammered home the concept of starting out slowly, so hopefully you haven't forgotten that point already. Spacing your runs out from each other by not doing back-to-back days (taking at least a day in between runs) is the same concept as taking walking breaks between running efforts. The breaks let your muscles and joints recover to keep you feeling good.

ENGINE VS. CHASSIS

Even if you're coming from another sport and have cardiovascular fitness (a strong engine), you'll still need to ease into running to give your musculoskeletal system (your chassis) time to ramp up.

Likewise, if you're coming from a strength-oriented sport like weightlifting, you'll have a strong chassis but need to ease into running to let your engine catch up.

INJURIES: ACUTE VS. CHRONIC

Flat-out, injuries suck. But a little knowledge about injuries and some tools to help manage them can help you move past them quicker. Know that injuries come in different forms:

acute • \ ə-'kyüt \ 1. *adj.* Not to be confused with "a cute" injury (no injuries are cute), acute injuries happen to you in one instance and cause sudden, sometimes severe pain. Also known as *traumatic injuries*—you fell and broke your wrist, for example, or you rubbed your heels raw with blisters.

chronic • \ 'krän-ik \ 1. *adj.* Not to be confused with the slang term for marijuana, this term is used to describe pain that's continual or occurring again and again. *Overuse injuries*, where certain soft tissues (or sometimes bones) become irritated from repetitive motion, fall into this category—your knee pain flares up if you run back-to-back days, your hip hurts when you run and don't do certain stretches.

Very important note: None of the following should be substituted for in-person medical advice.

TROUBLESHOOTING: ACUTE INJURIES

Here's a breakdown of acute injuries organized by what you did to yourself, what you can do about it, and how to prevent yourself from doing it again.

SPRAINED ANKLE

» **Oops:** Straining or actually spraining an ankle—you take a misstep on a curb, step on a rock or root, or get tripped up by your dog and roll your ankle.

» **Potential fix:** Good, old-fashioned "RICE": **rest** (take some time off from running until it feels strong enough); **ice** (ice your sore ankle for fifteen minutes at a time); **compression** (wrap the ice tightly around your ankle, and consider wearing compression socks when done icing to help encourage blood flow); **elevation** (put your foot up above your heart, like on a stack of pillows on the couch). In addition to RICE, do any exercises given to you by a physical therapist to help speed up healing.

» **Potential prevention:** Do the below exercises regularly to help strengthen ankles. Strengthening ankles can help ward off ankle sprains.

ANKLE-STRENGTHENING EXERCISES
- **Draw the alphabet:** Sit in a chair and pretend to draw the alphabet, A to Z with the toes of the injured foot. To make it harder, when you're done air-drawing all twenty-six letters, write it backward, Z to A.
- **Balance:** Stand on one foot and try to balance on it. To make this harder, stand on a pillow. To make it harder still, move the other leg to point toward imaginary positions on an imaginary clock on the ground in front of you: twelve o'clock, three o'clock, six o'clock, and nine o'clock, while balancing on the other leg. Switch legs and repeat.

There are more exercises for strengthening ankles and other body parts that use props like elastic bands you can get from physical therapists' offices or online, but for simplicity's sake, all the exercises in this book use just your body and the occasional household item.

STUBBED TOE

» **Oops:** Just as those dastardly curbs, rocks, and roots can cause an ankle roll, they can also cause you to stub your toe. A badly stubbed toe can actually break a bone or just become very sore and potentially turn a toenail black (and it might eventually fall off).

» **Potential fix:** RICE—and if it's not healing or really, really hurts, get an x-ray to rule out a broken bone.

» **Potential prevention:** Watch where you're going! Seems silly (and rude!), but since it's easy to zone out on a run, sometimes you just need to pay more attention to your footing. If you're trail running, focus on picking your feet up a little more than you normally do to avoid stubbing your toe because of shuffling. And, for sure if you're trail running and have a propensity for stubbing your toe, get yourself some trail running shoes that have a hearty rubber toe bumper. That chunk of rubber is there specifically for that reason.

BLISTERS

» **Oops:** Blisters happen as a result of heat, friction, moisture, or a combination of all three. They may seem little and like no big deal, but they suck and can make every step—while running or even walking—excruciating.

» **Potential fix:** If a blister develops during a run and you're not carrying a Band-Aid or duct tape (because, who does, unless you're on an epic mountain run?), you'll probably have to end your run and hobble home. When you do get home, you have two choices: leave the blister and wait until it goes down on its own—covering it with a Band-Aid, duct tape, or specific blister-care product—or pop it. To pop it, clean the area with antiseptic (rubbing alcohol works). Clean or burn the end of a needle. Puncture the blister, and gently push the liquid out. (Some sicko in your family might want to watch this, so invite them over before you do it.) Clean area again. Apply an antibacterial ointment and cover with a Band-Aid, but let it air out when sleeping to allow the skin to dry.

» **Potential prevention:** Wear good, well-fitting socks made of sweat-wicking material. Socks that are too large are major culprits of blistering due to bunching. Socks made of cotton are also culprits. Wear shoes that fit well. Too tight, too big, arch support hitting your foot in the wrong place—all culprits for blistering.

CHAFING

» **Oops:** Some item of clothing or accessory literally rubs you the wrong way, causing friction. Chafing is like blistering, but instead of a liquid-filled bubble, you get raw, red, sometimes oozing skin.

» **Potential fix:** If you're chafing on the run, try to adjust the item irritating you. Fold over a seam, take off a shirt, roll up a sleeve. If that doesn't work and you return home with shredded skin, bite your lower lip (because it'll hurt) and get in the shower or bath to clean off the area. Apply antibacterial ointment and cover with a bandage. Leave open when sleeping to allow skin to dry and heal.

» **Potential prevention:** Shop—and dress—wisely (refer to Chapter 4). If anything irritates your skin when you first put it on, know that's a recipe for chafing. If you know a certain part of your body is sensitive to chafing, apply a skin lubricant; Vaseline or products made specifically for anti-chafing will take away the friction that causes irritation.

BRUISES AND ABRASIONS

» **Oops:** If you trip for any reason on the run, or accidentally run into something, you could get a bruise or an abrasion—like a skinned knee.

» **Potential fix:** If your ego is also bruised, take it and your bruised self home. You'll both be fine. For an abrasion, treat it like you would chafed skin (see previous section).

» **Potential prevention:** These things happen, but if they happen often, consider revisiting your run specialty store to make sure you're in the best shoes for your gait (see page 60). Also, do the ankle-strengthening exercises and core exercises (see page 9) to help with balance. However, know that everyone trips once in a while, and sometimes there is nothing to blame/use to prevent it.

ICE VS. HEAT

Ice is used to fight inflammation and, generally speaking, should be used immediately following an acute injury in fifteen-minute increments spread out throughout the first forty-eight hours of an acute injury.

Heat encourages blood circulation and, generally speaking, should be used after forty-eight hours for an acute injury.

However, there are benefits to both, and some recommend using whichever feels better to your injury.

TROUBLESHOOTING: CHRONIC INJURIES

Chronic injuries are the ones that come back every so often to remind you of strains and muscle imbalances and to make you say to yourself, "Shoot. I should be doing those strengthening exercises my physical therapist told me to do." Here's a breakdown of the most common chronic injuries new runners tend to experience, broken down by how you can tell what might be ailing you, the potential cause(s) of the pain, what you can do about it, and how to prevent the pain from coming back.

> **Very important note, reiterated:** None of the following should be used in place of medical advice.

"MY KNEE HURTS RIGHT HERE."

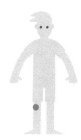

» **How so?** Your knee feels swollen, awkward, and/or like something is rubbing.

» **Might be:** "Runner's knee"/patellofemoral pain syndrome.

» **Why on earth:** Misalignment of bones from your hips to your feet; weakness or tightness in muscles from your quadriceps to your feet; overuse, especially combined with either of the first two reasons.

» **Potential fix:** RICE; anti-inflammatories; visit a running shoe store to assess your shoes (you may need a gait analysis and new shoes; see page 60); see a practitioner for a diagnosis and treatment plan to stretch and strengthen.

» **Potential prevention:** Actually do the stretching and strengthening exercises given to you by a practitioner. Try the following stretch, made famous by CrossFit trainer and author of *Becoming a Supple Leopard*, Kelly Starrett. "The typical person is already really tight in the quads and hip flexors from all the sitting we tend to do throughout the day," says Kirk Warner, a running coach for the online coaching website The Run Experience. This stretch can help combat that tightness and ward off knee pain.

COUCH STRETCH

1. Place a pillow or towel on the floor, close to and in front of a couch or wall. Facing away from the couch or wall, place your right knee on the pillow or towel and bring your right foot behind you (as if you're doing a standing quad stretch) and place the top of the right foot against the couch or wall with toes pointed.

2. Step forward with your left foot so it rests directly beneath the left knee and your leg makes a 90-degree angle. Lift your upper body so it's as upright as possible, trying to keep a flat back.

3. Hold for 1–2 minutes, feeling a deep stretch in your quad and hip flexor (don't forget to breathe, because this will hurt).

4. Switch sides and repeat.

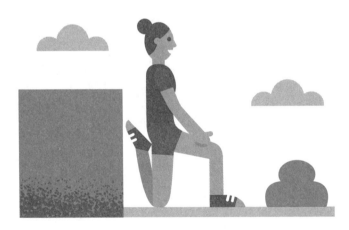

"MY KNEE HURTS RIGHT HERE."

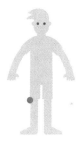

» **How so?** It hurts to bend your leg; pain is on the outside of your knee.

» **Might be:** Iliotibial band syndrome (ITBS)

» **Why on earth:** Muscle imbalances or tightness in the low back, pelvis, hips, glutes, and/or knees; unsupportive running shoes; repetitive use on uneven roads; anatomy issues.

» **Potential fix:** RICE; anti-inflammatories; foam rolling (see page 147); stretching. See a practitioner for a proper diagnosis and treatment plan.

» **Potential prevention:** Regularly strengthen and stretch hips, knees, and low back; strengthen core; use a foam roller regularly; wear good running shoes; actually do exercises given by practitioner.

STANDING ITB STRETCH

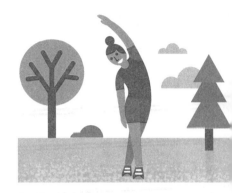

1. Stand with both feet flat on the floor and cross the leg of the knee that hurts behind your healthy leg so that the front of your injured knee is flush against the back of your healthy knee (let's assume at least one of your knees is healthy—if not, just repeat on the other side).

2. Place the hand of the same-side-as-your-injured-knee arm on your head, with your other hand resting on the hip of your healthy leg. Stretch your upper body toward the hand on your hip.

FIGURE 4 STRETCH

1. Lie on your back with your knees bent and feet flat on the floor. Place the ankle of your sore leg on the knee of your not-sore leg.

2. Reach your arms forward on either side of your not-sore leg and clasp your hands behind that leg.

3. Pull gently on that leg to feel the stretch in the outer butt muscles of your sore leg.

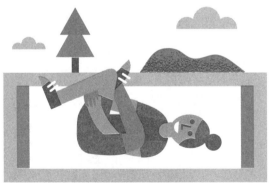

FOAM ROLL THE SHIT OUT OF IT

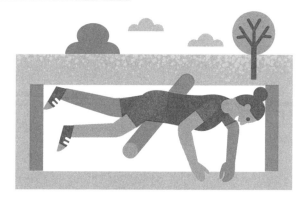

1. Lie with the outside of your quad resting (it won't feel like rest) on the foam roller and your hands on the ground supporting you for balance.

2. Use slow, long motions to roll your outer thigh back and forth on foam roller for 1–2 minutes, breathing.

IF IT HURTS TO ROLL, ROLL

"Knots and trigger points—or bumps and lumps—are normal in muscle tissue," says Boulder, Colorado–based physical therapist Charlie Merrill. "But when they're hypersensitive, it's a sign that that tissue is struggling to heal or normalize itself." The theory is that rolling will calm down that part of the tissue and desensitize and smooth it out before it becomes a bigger problem.

For how long should you roll? Merrill says to think about tenderizing a steak. "You're not gonna sit there and bang on it with a hammer for ten minutes because then it'll be flat, and it'll be on the grill and then taste like shit," he says. "You're just trying to bring blood flow to the area to create some movement and space to calm the nervous system, and you can do that in a couple of minutes."

"MY SHINS HURT."

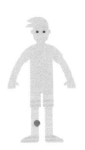

» **Might be:** Shin splints

» **How can you tell:** Sharp or dull/throbbing pain in one or both of your shins, either when running/walking or after, or from touching the sore spot.

» **Why on earth:** Overuse, often from increasing activity too drastically (i.e., going from zero to sixty on a training plan); having flat feet or tight muscles in the feet; old, worn-down shoes.

» **Potential fix:** RICE; anti-inflammatories; stretching; seeing a practitioner for a proper diagnosis and for prescribed stretches.

» **Potential prevention:** Wear good shoes; slowly ease into running (see Chapter 6); strengthen feet by walking barefoot, doing exercises (see next page).

CALF STRETCHES

STRETCH 1

1. Stand facing a wall, with one leg behind the other and your hands placed flat against the wall.

2. Lean in to the wall, keeping your back leg straight while bending the front leg. (The stretch is at the back of the back leg.) Hold for 30 seconds.

3. Repeat 2–3 times, and switch legs.
This stretches the gastrocnemius muscle in your calf, which can be tight enough to strain your shin muscles and cause pain on the front of your leg.

STRETCH 2

1. Bend the back leg slightly, and repeat the above steps. You may have to move your back leg closer to your front leg to do this.
This stretches the soleus muscle, which can also contribute to the pain in the front of your leg.

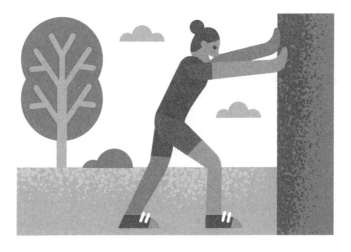

TOE RAISES

1. Sit with both feet flat on the floor and your knees bent to 90 degrees.

2. Slowly raise the toes of one of your feet.

3. Slowly lower. (Start with just a few repetitions and build up to more.)

4. Repeat on the other leg or do both legs together.

"MY FOOT HURTS."

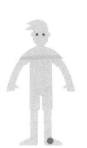

» **Might be:** Plantar fasciitis

» **How can you tell:** Your heel and/or arch of your foot hurts, especially first thing in the morning; pain may ease up with walking or running, then return once you stop.

» **Why on earth:** Stiff ankles; old, worn-out shoes; ramping up running too fast.

» **Potential fix:** RICE; see a practitioner for a diagnosis and a treatment plan; stretching.

CALF STRETCH (PAGE 149)

GOLF BALL MASSAGE

1. Sit with knees bent and feet flat on the floor and a golf ball in front of you on the floor. Roll the bottom of the foot in pain on the golf ball, giving the muscles in your foot a massage. Roll the other foot, just because it feels good (and can help prevent the same fate as your hurt foot).

» **Potential prevention:** Ease into running. Don't increase mileage too fast. (See page 112.)

» **Night splint:** There are contraptions for sale online or in drugstores that splint your lower leg but hold your foot in a flexed position while you sleep. These are used to treat plantar fasciitis.

WHEN TO GET NEW SHOES

Running in old shoes can actually cause injuries and make existing injuries worse. Experts say you need new running shoes every three hundred to five hundred miles or about every six months. But if you're not logging every run or every mile you walk in your running shoes—through grocery store aisles or while purposely exercising—how do you know how many total miles you've accumulated? And since there's a wide range in how often people run and how much wear and tear each person puts on a shoe with each run, how do you know when you need a new pair? A few telltale signs:

- Your shoes aren't new, and a few body parts that don't usually bother you start hurting.

- The cushioning feels different—compressed or flat—from when the shoes were new.

- The outsole shows breakdown in one part over the other.

- The upper has holes in it, which means the shoe isn't supporting your foot like it used to.

STOMACH ISSUES

Some ailments aren't classified as acute or chronic, but they suck nonetheless. Stomach issues can happen on the run (cue poop puns here). Causes of gastrointestinal (GI) distress while running can range from dehydration to irritation from anti-inflammatories to eating a cheeseburger thirty minutes before your run.

Solving stomach issues requires some trial and error with what you ingest in the hours surrounding your run. If issues persist, see a doctor.

THE DOCTOR WILL SEE YOU NOW

Do not (repeat, do *not*) use only this book to diagnose and treat your ailments. Use it as a guide, sure, and a helpful one at that. But for a professional diagnosis and treatment plan for an acute injury, chronic injury, or persistent stomach issues, see a medical practitioner of some sort.

Finding a practitioner who specializes in running injuries will be your best form of defense from paying someone to say this: "If it hurts when you run, don't run."

PRACTITIONERS, DEFINED

» **General practitioner.** A well-rounded doctor whom you see for everything from strep throat to a sharp pain in your knee and who may refer you to a specialist.

» **Orthopedic doctor.** A doctor specializing in the musculoskeletal system—your bones and muscles.

» **Chiropractor.** A licensed health care professional who moves your bones and sometimes uses tools to treat muscles.

» **Physical therapist.** A licensed health care professional who addresses pains with treatment and stretching and strengthening exercises. Sometimes treats with dry needling—sticking tiny needles in your muscles to help them release.

» **Acupuncturist.** A professional who works on muscles with very tiny needles in specific places, based on Eastern medicine. Sometimes uses/prescribes herbs.

» **Massage therapist.** A professional who works on muscles and occasionally alignment with their hands to help you feel gooood. Can be great for recovery.

» **Rolfer.** A professional who takes massage to the next level by lifting your muscles away from your bones for structural integration.

» **Prolotherapist.** A professional who uses injections to purposefully re-injure weak ligaments so they tighten up and hold bones in place.

This is a small sampling of the types of practitioners available for various ailments, but they are arguably the most common for running-specific needs.

THE COMEBACK PLAN

If you do suffer an acute or chronic injury, return to running gradually and carefully. Take a step back and start up again, alternating running and walking as you did when you first started running, increasing the time running if—and only if—your body says you should. "Some pain when returning to running is normal," explains Merrill. "Your tissues will be getting used to running again. If those pains subside during your run, and don't increase after your run, you should be okay to continue your return to running. But be sure to listen to your body."

SELF-HELP

Seeing a doctor or other medical professional is great (and oftentimes necessary for treating an injury), but it's also beneficial—physically and mentally—to leave any appointment feeling like your injury is somewhat in your control. The following aren't save-all, miracle cures, but having these tools in your arsenal can help.

FOAM ROLLING

A tube of dense foam will become your best friend (because it can alleviate a multitude of woes) but also your frenemy (because it hurts like a bitch). Use it for self-massage, rolling out tight muscles like your iliotibial band (see page 145), quadriceps, low back, calves, and more. And use it to stretch your upper back and chest (see page 101). You may be amazed at how much pain this seemingly innocuous foam cylinder can inflict, but it is all good pain . . . really good pain that is helpful in keeping you healthy. (See page 147 for how long to roll.)

There are a whole host of foam rollers made of different densities of foam on the market. They range from smooth to somewhat bumpy to downright pokey, with protrusions of dense foam digging into your muscles as you roll around in super-beneficial self-torture. Smooth rollers will allow the most versatility for various stretches, while bumpy rollers better replicate thumbs of strong masseuses.

STRETCHING/MOBILITY

The jury is currently out on whether regular stretching is good for a runner, but many running coaches are pro "mobility," which is a combination of light, dynamic stretching and rolling.

Doing web searches for, say, "hip mobility for runners," produces online videos you can follow in the comfort of your own living room, but attending exercise classes, signing up for online coaching, or hiring a strength and mobility coach of your own can help safely guide you through mobility exercises that will keep your parts working smoothly. These exercises may have you reaching for a foam roller, lacrosse ball, massage ball, stick, band, or other prop that will stretch, strengthen, or massage your muscles.

CROSS-TRAINING

Cross-training simply means other active physical activities running. Some cross-training activities—like hiking and cycling—use some of the same muscles as running, while others—like rock climbing—give your running muscles a break and help build functional strength. Cross-training on days in between running days, or when an ache is giving you a check-engine light when you run, is a great way to stay active while still heeding the warning that you need a break from running. For more on cross-training, see Chapter 6.

Sucky thought zapped by this chapter:

"Running always hurts."

"I don't want to eat gel."

FUEL

(A.K.A. WHAT TO EAT AND DRINK SO RUNNING SUCKS LESS)

Now that you're running, you're hungry like the wolf. If you have a few bad eating habits, consider *keeping* a couple of them while starting a running program. If you go on a diet or cut out your favorite food/drink *while* starting to run, you're bound to associate running with the *suckiness* that is not having your favorite food(s)/drink(s).

That said, becoming a runner who loves running will likely make you want to alter some unhealthy eating/drinking habits.

Not that you're running solely to lose weight (run for fun), but if you're curious, running burns roughly one hundred calories a mile, though that number can vary drastically—it's higher the more a person weighs, the less efficient they are, the faster they're running, and the hillier the terrain.

WHY DO NEW RUNNERS GAIN WEIGHT?

Many people start running and are shocked that they gain weight initially before losing. One explanation is perception: "I'm running now, so I can eat more," which is sort of true but can get out of hand, as many people overestimate the number of calories running burns. Another explanation is that *since* they're running, they're hungrier and therefore eating more. With both reasons, if calories burned don't exceed calories ingested, weight loss doesn't happen. The takeaway? If one of your goals is to lose weight, pay attention to what you eat.

Another reason for weight gain is that body composition changes with any new exercise regimen . . . and muscle weighs more than fat. You'll feel stronger with your new pastime of running, so forget the numbers on the scale and revel in your new strength.

PROOF THAT RUNNING DOESN'T SUCK

This is how many miles it will take to burn off some common foods.

Food	Burn it off in:
Donut	2 miles
Slice of pizza	3 miles
Giant burrito	9 miles
Scoop of ice cream	1–2 miles
Pint carton of ice cream	7–8 miles
IPA beer	2 miles
Guinness	1–2 miles
Bottle of wine	6 miles

> **KEY NO. 8 TO MAKING RUNNING NOT SUCK: FUEL WISELY**
>
> The more care you give yourself regarding what you put in your mouth, the less sucky running will feel. This does not mean you have to entirely change how you eat to enjoy running. Rather, paying attention to what you ingest before, during, and after your run will make a difference in how much running sucks or doesn't.

MORE THAN GEL

Back to that reason you said you don't want to become a runner: "I don't want to eat gel."

Gels (which are made up mostly of the simple sugars glucose and fructose) are fantastic mid-run because they digest easily and absorb quickly into your body to give you energy. But that doesn't mean you *have* to eat them.

"There are so many options when it comes to fueling your run," says Claire Shorenstein, certified running coach and founder of EatforEndurance.com. "No one is forcing you to eat things that you don't like. It may take a while to figure out which foods you enjoy that also don't upset your stomach, but trial and error will help you do that."

So you don't barf, burp excessively, or bonk[1] on your run . . . all actions that would make running undeniably *sucky*, this section will guide you toward good options for what and when to eat in relation to your run.

NUTRITION FACTS

You know these words, but here's why they matter to you as a runner:

» **Carbohydrates:** What your body burns, mostly, for energy while running and living.

---

1 **bonk** \ 'bäŋk \ 1. *verb.* To seriously and drastically run out of energy mid-run, so much so that you feel like you just can't take another step. Also known as "hitting the wall."

» **Fats:** What your body relies on to lubricate your joints, to help absorb nutrients, and to keep you satiated.

» **Farts:** What comes out of you if you eat too much fat and protein before a run.

» **Protein:** What your body relies on to repair muscles and satiate you better than nonprotein foods.

» **Salt/Sodium:** What you lose when you sweat. It's also essential for avoiding cramping, sending nerve impulses throughout our bodies, and regulating dehydration.

» **Vitamins:** Essential for growth and overall health—energy, metabolism, as antioxidants, to absorb nutrients, and so on—and runners need more of them than non-runners since you lose them through sweat.

» **Minerals:** Essential for growth and overall health, and runners need more of them than non-runners. For example, the mineral iron helps form new red blood cells (which break down when running) to help maintain energy.

WHAT RUNNERS NEED TO KNOW ABOUT FAT

Our bodies tap into easily available calories (ingested carbs) and proteins for energy before they tap into fat stores, but runners can get their bodies to start using up fat cells by running for longer (which you will do eventually), adding intensity (whether running or cross-training), or running regularly (increased frequency helps your body tap into fat stores).

NUTRITION, A.K.A. FOOD

Nutrition is what runners, cyclists, triathletes, and other athletes tend to call food when they're nerding out. The term *nutrition* makes food sound more serious, and when you're running, cycling, or training regularly in any way, what you put in your body *is* more serious because it directly impacts your experience in your sport.

The act of running jostles stomachs up and down enough to make what you ingest before and during a run really matter. What you eat and drink afterward has more to do with recovering well to feel good the rest of the day and the next.

PRE-RUN FUEL

What you eat before the run affects how much energy you have during the run and how much or little you feel like barfing, pooping, burping, or spitting during your run.

Know that everyone's body reacts differently to foods, so getting used to what to eat and how far ahead of a run you should eat it will have to be dialed in by trial and error.

» **Trial:** You eat a burrito one hour before an afternoon run.

» **Error:** You feel as if you're carrying a burrito baby in your gut and therefore can hardly pick up your feet (and are burping cilantro and chicken).

» **Solution:** Eat a burrito two hours or more before a run, or eat something smaller, like a taco or a half a burrito (or a plain bagel or some energy chews) an hour before.

~~~~~~~~~~

» **Trial:** You don't eat anything before a 9:00 a.m. run.

» **Error:** Every rock looks like an egg, and every pothole looks like a giant waffle, and you're drooling. Plus, you have so little energy that you have to walk home, and you might feel light-headed as you do so.

» **Solution:** Eat a carb-rich snack, such as a half of a plain waffle, a banana, or a couple of bites of your kid's pancake thirty to sixty minutes before your run.

~~~~~~~~~~~~~~~~~~~~

» **Tip:** If you've decided to run first thing in the morning but have a hard time eating anything before your run, load up the night before. Have a dinner later than usual or a snack before bed. The energy you store at night will help fuel you through your morning run if you'd rather eat breakfast afterward.

WHEN TO EAT

A general rule for how long before a run to eat is this: wait two hours to run after a big meal; wait thirty minutes to one hour (or longer) to run after eating a small snack. That doesn't guarantee that a hamburger, fries, pickles, and coleslaw will sit perfectly in your gut on an evening run two hours after you ate it. Nor does it guarantee that taking a few bites of a plain pancake ten minutes before a morning run will cause problems. Trial and error will help you figure out what works for you.

Simple carbohydrates are a lot easier for your gut to digest than complex carbs or fatty foods.

simple carbohydrates · \ ˈsim-pəl car-bo-hy-drāt-es \ 1. *noun.* Foods that are far less likely to make you barf while running; for example, fruit without much fiber (like bananas) or refined carbs (like white bread). Generally easier to digest than complex carbohydrates before or during your run.

complex carbohydrates · \ ˈkäm-ˌpleks car-bo-hy-drāts\ 1. *noun.* Foods that have more of a complex makeup and therefore take longer to digest, which can make you have to make excessive bathroom stops while running. Complex carbs (like lentil stew) are generally better for you but may not be the best choice before or during a run. But then again, they may be fine, depending on the individual.

EASY-TO-DIGEST PRE-RUN SNACKS

Here are some ideas of easy-to-digest, simple carbohydrate, pre-run snacks:

- Plain bagel, waffle, toast, or pancake (white is easier to digest than wheat, oat, or multigrain)

- Banana

- One serving (usually half a bag) of energy chews, which are like gummy bears for endurance athletes

- Dried fruit (not too much, or it'll stop you up or cause the opposite problem if very fibrous)

MID-RUN FUEL

Unless you haven't eaten in days or are running more than an hour, you probably don't need to eat mid-run.

But if either of the above is true, simple carbohydrates in super-easy-to-digest forms will be your best bet. This is where energy gels come in very handy. Though gooey and not all that appealing, the viscous consistency of an energy gel makes it easy to ooze right down your throat and start working its energy-giving magic right away. A ham sandwich or a handful of pretzels will not go down as easily as food engineered specifically to be easy to digest, like a gel or energy chew.

Still, there will be some trial and error for what works for you mid-run (again, if you're out for an hour or more or are starting out with an empty tank). As you'll read in Chapter 10, it's never a good idea to try out a gel or chew—or any "fuel"—for the first time during a race, unless you want to live on the edge and risk pooping your pants in front of hundreds of other people (in the somewhat rare event the gel or chew really doesn't sit well with you).

» **Trial:** You try to ingest an energy gel during a long run/walk.

» **Error:** You squeeze the packet too vigorously and mostly miss your mouth, sending viscous gel cascading down your arm.

» **Solution:** Slow to a walk until you get good at this: Tear open gel packet with your teeth (keeping top part of wrapper attached or putting it in your pocket so you don't litter), squeeze a small amount of gel into your mouth until you become advanced and can squeeze and ingest a whole packet at once.

» **Trial:** You try to eat an energy chew while running hard.

» **Error:** The bag explodes when you open it on the run. When you recover a chew from the asphalt to put in your mouth, the cube-shaped gummy gets lodged in your throat and you have to flag down a passerby to give you the Heimlich maneuver.

» **Solution:** Open the bag before your run and stow the chews in a pocket or belt, or slow to a walk to both open it and to eat them.

HOW TO CARRY FOOD ON THE RUN

Maybe your running shorts, tights, or pants have a pocket large enough for a gel or a few energy chews you've put in a baggie. If not, waist-mounted storage options exist that can carry your fuels as well as your phone, money, and/or keys. Also, hydration systems—like a handheld water bottle—often have pockets to stash other items like gels or chews. And if you're using liquid energy, you'll need a way to carry liquids anyway, so look for an option with pockets for other items. (For more on this, see Chapter 4.)

"Running retooled my approach to diet and lifestyle. I no longer thought of food as something I needed to just keep me alive or finish the next workout. Food is now the essential catalyst for performance and health."

—Scott Jurek, 7-time Western States 100-Mile Endurance Run winner and author of *Eat and Run: My Unlikely Journey to Ultramarathon Greatness* and *North: Finding My Way While Running the Appalachian Trail*

EASY-TO-DIGEST MID-RUN SNACKS

The following are formulated to be quick and easy to digest while your stomach is being bounced up and down by your running steps:

- **ENERGY GEL:** Gooey, viscous gel in an on-the-go packet. Comes in a variety of flavors from multiple brands.

- **ENERGY CHEW:** Gummy bears (though not bear-shaped) for endurance athletes, formulated with simple sugars and fruit flavoring. Come in a variety of flavors from multiple brands.

- **LIQUID ENERGY:** Water mixed with powder or premixed to deliver calories in a liquid form. Comes in a variety of flavors from multiple brands.

POST-RUN FUEL

The most beneficial food items following a run are protein-rich foods that aid muscle recovery and replenish calories burned. The general rule of thumb is that ingesting protein-rich foods within thirty minutes of exercise will give your body the most benefit.

Post-run food and drink is, like anything, trial and error.

» **Trial:** You chug a beer upon returning home from your run, thinking you're "hydrating" and also "refueling" because, you know, wheat.

» **Error:** It tastes so good, you have four more and feel like shit the next day.

» **Solution:** Chug a glass of water and some salty nuts before you drink that beer. Or double-fist with beer and water, putting one down occasionally to snack on said nuts. The water will rehydrate you better and fill you up so you have three more beers instead of four. And the salt (electrolytes!) and nuts (protein!) will aid your recovery.

» **Trial:** You get distracted with work, kids, laundry, or whatever upon returning from your run and don't remember to eat until two hours later.

» **Error:** You get so hangry (hungry + angry) that you yell at everyone around you and want to eat everything in sight, all at once. And you feel awful—sore and depleted—the rest of that day and the next.

» **Solution:** Make sure you eat something carb- and protein-rich within thirty or so minutes of finishing your run.

PROTEIN-RICH POST-RUN FOODS

Protein is known to help muscles recover and to help satiate a hungry runner. Not all protein-rich foods go down easy after a workout, so here are some suggestions for good options for runners:

- Chocolate milk (or strawberry, or vanilla . . . the sugar helps you recover, too)
- Protein bar
- Protein shake/smoothie
- Peanut butter sandwich
- Eggs

HYDRATION, A.K.A. DRINKS

Hydration is what runners and other athletes call water, sports drinks, and other liquids when they're nerding out and what said liquids do for a body while running (as in "I hydrated, and so I peed").

The same jostling that can make it hard to ingest food on the run can also make it a challenge to ingest the right amount of liquid, and figuring out the right amount for you on any given day—pre-, mid-, and post-run—is, you guessed it, trial and error. But there are some guidelines that will help.

» **Trial:** You didn't bring any liquids on a run in 105° temps.

» **Error:** You felt terrible; plus, your face was white with the sodium your body expelled through sweat when you got home.

» **Solution:** Hydrate better before your run, the night/day before your run, and consider bringing a small hydration system containing a sports drink with sodium on your run.

» **Trial:** You carried a full hydration pack on a 5K fun run.

» **Error:** Your back hurt, your legs hurt, your lungs hurt, and you finished your run with a full hydration pack because there were aid stations handing out water every half mile.

» **Solution:** Don't carry a hydration pack at a 5K with aid stations.

Some more tips:
- If you are dying of thirst on a run, drink more water before your run, even the night before or generally throughout the day.
- If your belly sloshes during a run, focus on hydration throughout the day or night before your run and avoid chugging water right before.
- If you're covered in white, dried sweat after your run, drink more water and/ or hydration mix with electrolytes before or during your run or in general throughout the day.

TYPES OF DRINKS SUITABLE FOR RUNNERS

WATER

The basis for all hydration, also for . . . life; hydrates your body's cells; doesn't stink up a bottle or make it moldy if left a few days unwashed; is available from drinking fountains sometimes found on running route; doesn't usually upset stomachs.

ELECTROLYTE/SPORTS DRINK

Usually formulated with helpful minerals—like sodium—that can help sustain energy while hydrating you; some contain a lot of sugar that you don't need, so read labels (a small amount of sugar can help give you energy but isn't necessary).

JUICE

Liquid fruit, sometimes with added sugar; can be nice to have after a run in a smoothie; can make you sick if ingested before— or especially during—a run.

COFFEE/TEA

Caffeinated (or not) and therefore can jump-start a run; can also help get bowels moving before a run.

Caffeine used to be thought of as the Great Dehydrator, but that has been largely disproven. In fact, the current school of thought regarding caffeine is that it can increase endorphins, help you enjoy your run more by making you mentally alert . . . and simply wake you the hell up so you can get out the door on a morning run. For some people (but not everyone), caffeine even helps process energy more efficiently. The downsides of caffeine are that too much can make you jittery, and it can mess with your stomach on a run if you're not used to it. But generally speaking, studies have shown that up to 550 mg, or five cups of coffee, is okay. However, drinking five cups of coffee before a run can have you jittery as all get-out, or worse, desperate for a public bathroom, or ten.

DAIRY DRINKS

Unless you like making milkshakes that come out of your mouth, save dairy drinks for after a run (when the protein can aid recovery).

ALCOHOL

Can make you run in a zigzag pattern (or barf) if ingested before a run, so not advised; can make you more dehydrated if ingested the night before a run; can taste great after a run (fresh, cold beer, in particular); beer, being around 90 percent water, can rehydrate; carbs in beer can also help you recover. Just take it easy, tiger!

SMOOTHIES

Since smoothies can be packed with liquid (water, juice, dairy), nutrients (fruits and vegetables), and sometimes proteins (powders, nut butters), they can be fantastic recovery drinks; can project out of your mouth during a run (like milkshakes) if ingested pre-run without enough time to digest.

RECOVERY/PROTEIN MIXES

Protein is key in helping muscles rebuild and recover. It helps you feel good the rest of the day after a run and the days to follow, so recovery drinks and protein mixes (powders mixed with water, or sometimes milk or other liquids) can be a really handy way to ingest protein after a run.

PRE-RUN HYDRATION

Like a plant, and every living thing, you need to be watered to thrive. Pre-hydrating—and hydrating well throughout your running and non-running days—will help you have a full tank anytime you do head out on a run. Chugging a glass of water within an hour of heading out on a run won't serve you well; your belly will slosh, you'll have to stop to pee, and you'll feel crappy overall. Instead, make sure you're hydrated all the time, and take small sips of water leading up to your run.

> **Tip:** If you're running first thing in the morning, or the forecast looks particularly hot for the next day, hydrate well the day and night before.

MID-RUN HYDRATION

Unless you're running more than forty-five minutes or so, it's notably hot and humid, or you're super dehydrated from a big bender the night before, you won't need to carry water or a sports drink on your run. But if any of the aforementioned is true, see page 79 for hydration-carrying devices, and follow these tips:

- Take sips rather than chugs.
- Drink before you're thirsty.
- Don't pound water, thinking you're being a great hydrator.[2]

WHAT ARE ELECTROLYTES?

We lose electrolytes (essentially, salt) through sweat, and they need to be replaced to keep us from falling over. Electrolytes help keep cells healthy and functioning properly, and they spark nerve impulses to help control how our bodies process vitamins, minerals, and waste. Most people not working out for extended periods of time get enough electrolytes in their daily diet if they eat things like bananas, watermelon, and pickles, but if you increase your exercise level, you may also need to increase your electrolyte intake.

2   See hyponatremia sidebar on page 173.

WHAT IS HYPONATREMIA, AND WHY SHOULD YOU CARE?

Maybe you've heard headlines about how runners have died in marathons from drinking too much water. Hyponatremia, though statistically rare, happens when the bloodstream becomes diluted by H_2O and there isn't enough sodium and potassium. You generally don't have to worry about it unless you start running long distances and pounding water, but be aware of its dangers, and balance out your water intake with foods rich in sodium and/or electrolyte drinks.

POST-RUN HYDRATION

Sometimes you'll finish a run and dive for a water, sports drink, or beer. Those days should tell you that you could afford to hydrate better before your run or bring water with you on a run.

If you're not thirsty after a run, though, that doesn't mean you shouldn't drink; rehydrating post-run will help aid your recovery. You'll feel much better the rest of the day and the next if you rehydrate quickly after a run than if you wait until you're parched.

The following are valuable liquids to choose from:

- **Water.** Replaces fluids lost while running. Keeps cells healthy.
- **Electrolyte/sports drink.** Replaces fluids, sodium, electrolytes, vitamins, and minerals, depending on the ingredients. Careful, though—these drinks can contain more sugar than you need. (For this reason, seek out brands that have all the good stuff and zero sugar.)
- **Coconut water.** Replaces electrolytes without added sugar. Currently very trendy.
- **Chocolate milk.** Replaces fluids, carbohydrates, and protein. (Also contains sugar.)
- **Protein drink.** Replaces protein (duh!) and often other vitamins and minerals while also replacing fluids.
- **Beer.** See page 171.

FIND YOUR SWEAT RATE BY PEEING

If you really want to get nerdy and find out how much you, and specifically you, need to drink/hydrate for a run and after, do this test:

1. Get naked, pee (or pee and then get naked), weigh yourself, and write down your weight.[3]
2. Go for a run, get naked again, weigh yourself again, write down your weight. If you urinate during your run, do the test another day.[4]
3. Do this math: 1 pound lost = 16 ounces fluid lost.

For example, if you lost 2 pounds during your run and you didn't drink anything on the run, you lost 32 ounces of fluids and need to replace that much to feel normal.

If you lost 2 pounds during your run and drank 4 ounces during your run, you lost 28 ounces (2 × 16 ounces = 32 ounces, minus 4 ounces) and need to replace that much to feel normal.

---

3 Doing this first thing in the morning will give you the most accurate reading.
4 If you drink during your run, add the amount to the amount of fluids lost.

Sucky thought zapped by this chapter:

"Running—and stuff runners eat—makes me barf."

"Runners are d-bags."

ETIQUETTE, THANK YOU VERY MUCH

It may seem like there's a certain code of conduct among runners, and, in many ways, there is. It can be intimidating when you don't know whether or not it's okay to spit when running with a partner (it is), what to do when you have to pee mid-run (you pee), or if it's okay to jaywalk/run (it depends).

KEY NO. 9 TO MAKING RUNNING NOT SUCK: BE NICE.

If you think all runners are nerds, d-bags, a-holes, or just part of some club that you don't know how to join—or don't want to—don't worry. Living by the golden rule and generally being nice will make you fit right in (and better the world while you're at it).

HOW TO NOT BECOME
THAT GUY OR GAL

You probably don't like that guy or gal in your office very much . . . the one who brags about their marathon or half marathon or throws numbers like 70.3[1] around as if people should know what they're talking about.

You will likely—and should—be excited about the sport you're beginning to love, but here's the easiest way to avoid sounding like a d-bag: don't talk about it unless you're asked. For example:

You: *I can't go out tonight.*

Coworker/friend: *Why not?*

You: *I'm gonna get up at 5:00 a.m.*

Coworker/friend: *Why on earth?*

You: *I started running a couple of weeks ago, and I really like going early. Do you want to come?*

. . . is better than this:

You: *I can't go out tonight because I'm getting up at 5:00 a.m. to go for a run, and my God, doesn't that make me sound virtuous and better than you?*

Be excited about it, but don't rub it in other people's faces. Rather, gently and enthusiastically recruit them to your new world, and you may just have some new running partners.

~~~~~~~~~~~~~~~~~~~~~~~

Read on to find out how to handle yourself on your runs in and among runners and non-runners alike.

....

1. The term 70.3 comes from the total number of miles covered in a half-Ironman triathlon between the swim (1.2), bike (56) and run (13.1).

BODILY FUNCTIONS

Running adds a whole new level of acceptability as far as bodily functions in company are concerned. Here's a look at all of them, plus how to make them even more acceptable on the run/walk.

BURPING
Bouncing up and down while you run can make the air inside you want to come up and out. Eating certain foods before a run can increase this.

Acceptable in running company?

FARTING
That jostling also can stir up your insides, keep you regular, and yes, make you fart. Some runners toot unapologetically. Some blame frogs for the noise and dogs for the smell. Others hang back from their running partners or groups and blow inconspicuously.

Acceptable in company?

Depends on the company, how you choose to do it, and if those two things align.

BLOWING SNOT ROCKETS
A runny, or clogged, nose is a drag on a run, as breathing freely is key to enjoyable running. And running can cause or increase an already runny nose since breathing heavily—especially in cold weather—makes the nose go into overdrive as the humidifier to your lungs. Instead of wiping your running snot on your sleeve, learn to blow a hearty snot rocket. Here's a step-by-step guide:

1. Slow your pace, maybe even to a walk.

2. Plug the less-clogged nostril with your index finger.

3. Turn your head toward the clogged nostril, and crane your head away from your body and down toward the ground (but, most importantly, away from your body and others'). While turned, make sure no runners are approaching on the snot side.

4. Take a big inhalation through your mouth, then close your mouth and blow the bejesus out the open nostril.

5. Repeat on the other side.

Acceptable in company?
Yes, as all runners need to do this. Just make sure you aim far, far away from anyone.

PEEING

Inevitably, you'll have to pee while on a run. You'll either get lucky and find one of the following:

» **Public restroom**, such as in a park or coffee shop

» **Open portable restroom**, such as at a construction site

» **Or you'll have to find a large tree**, dense bushes, or something that covers you. See sidebar on how.

Acceptable in company?
If you're not running alone, drop back from your partner or partners to become alone, and hide yourself. How well you hide yourself depends on your company and your general whereabouts.

PEEING IN PUBLIC, BY GENDER

Men undeniably have it easier, standing behind anything wider than their . . . part, to quickly whip it out and pee.

Men can also kneel down and pretend to tie a shoe, peeing out the bottom of their shorts.

Women have more maneuvering to do and more parts to bare . . .

. . . unless they're wearing shorts or a skirt and can pull off the move of squatting down, pulling the crotch of their shorts or skirt liner to the side, and peeing out the bottom.

Tip: To minimize the possibility of peeing on your shoes or suffering from splattering pee, use a wide stance, slightly stagger your feet, and pee on soft (read: permeable) surfaces as opposed to rock slabs.

POOPING

Having to poop while running happens because of the jostling that creates gas and . . . movement. The list of ideal places to poop is shorter than for peeing. Basically, find a public restroom or a open portable toilet, or wait until you get home (even if you have to slow to a walk).

Acceptable in company?

No one ever wants to see anyone else poop.

> **Tip:** If you know you often have to poop when you run, plan routes by restrooms, such as through public parks, past coffee shops, or construction sites with Porta-Potties.

WORST-CASE SCENARIO: HOW TO POOP IN THE WOODS

The Leave No Trace Center for Outdoor Ethics recommends the following methods for pooping in the woods.[2]

1. Make sure you're at least two hundred feet (seventy big steps) from a body of water (river, creek, lake, etc.).
2. Find a stick or sharp rock to dig a hole six to eight inches deep.
3. Do your thing (and good luck; consider leaning against a large rock, log, or tree for support).
4. Wipe with a leaf (preferably not poison oak or ivy, or stinging nettles) or flat rock.
5. Bury it (leaf or flat rock included), and bury it well.

SOCIAL INTERACTIONS

The following answers to common questions will help you negotiate social interactions as a runner.

RUN ETIQUETTE: ONE PARTNER/SMALL GROUP

» **Q:** How long should you wait for your running partner to show up?

» **A:** Follow these guidelines:

After five minutes: Text them, asking if you're in the right meeting place.

After ten minutes: Text them something snarky.

After fifteen minutes: Sayonara, partner. You have places to go.

....

2   Only do this in the woods, where the ground is soft enough to dig. *Do not do this in an urban area.*

Etiquette tip: Be on time yourself, or get ready for a passive-aggressive text, followed by a snarky text, followed by getting left behind.

» **Q:** Should I wear headphones while running with a partner, small group, or large group?

» **A:** Hell no.

STRETCHING AROUND OTHERS

Guys, if you must stretch in a group environment, wear shorts with built-in compression shorts. Women, wear longer shorts, shorts with compression shorts, or capris. Do not tell yourself that no one's looking (they are) or that no one can see anything (they can, and they don't want to).

RUN ETIQUETTE: LARGE GROUP

» **Q:** Should I run three or four abreast in a group, so we can all discuss *The Bachelor*?

» **A:** No. Run two abreast or less, depending on the width of the path. Running two by two still allows for discussions of hot topics like climate change and which bachelorette got sent home on the last episode.

» **Q:** Should a faster group drop a slower runner?

» **A:** No. No runner left behind.

» **Q:** Should I race my fellow runners on a casual group run?

» **A:** Not if you want to keep friends/running partners—or unless it's decided from the get-go that you're racing or sprinting at the end of a run for fun.

HITTING ON PEOPLE IN RUNNING CLUBS/ON GROUP RUNS

Plenty of people meet their mates in running clubs (see page 87)—but don't be creepy. As in life, take the hint and turn the conversation squarely back to running or small talk if someone is clearly uninterested. (Don't be that girl or guy who pounces on every attractive fellow runner, peppering them with clear pickup lines or requests for personal info. No one wants that person in their running group.)

ON THE ROAD

Sharing the road with other runners, walkers, babies, kids, cars, bikes, unicycles, Rollerbladers, and the like can be harmonious and safe. Here's how to politely and graciously get along with others:

» **Do:** Make a little noise by coughing or sniffing when approaching from behind. If the party ahead of you doesn't hear you or doesn't make enough room for you to pass by, politely say something like "Hi" or "Morning" as you approach. Follow that up with "Excuse me" or "Can I get by you?"

   This is more polite than yelling "*On your left!*" However, you can resort to saying that phrase gently and nicely if you need to, followed by "Thank you" and/or "Have a nice day."

» **Don't:** Be a jerk.

What if you get passed by other runners or walkers, including people pushing baby joggers, pregnant runners or walkers, walkers wearing casts, or kids?

» **Do:** Move to the far right of the sidewalk, path, or road and let them pass. It's okay to say something like "Good job."

» **Don't:** Worry about it, feel badly about yourself, or give up. Don't say anything too self-sabotaging, like "Way to make me feel slow," unless you can say it with a smile in your voice, on your face, and in your heart. (Yes, in your heart.) Saying negative things about ourselves, even when we're joking, can have negative effects on confidence. Rest assured, even the fastest runners out there get passed sometimes. Being pregnant or pushing a baby jogger doesn't slow parents down as much as you'd think it would. So be gracious and happy for them, and don't feel badly about yourself.

RUNNER VS. LOCALS

When running in a foreign country, or even a different city, remember that you're the foreigner and be cognizant of local cultures. Know whether it's culturally appropriate to wear certain types of running clothes, and bring money for coffee/tea and local baked goods on your way back to your hotel from a morning run. Yes, this is self-serving, but it's etiquette in that you're supporting the local economy. It also means you have cash to hail a cab or take public transport in the event you get lost and don't speak the language.

RUNNER VS. CAR

This combination is, potentially, the most dangerous. Follow these guidelines to keep everyone safe and happy:

» **Do:** Look drivers in the eye. When crossing streets in crosswalks, it's a good idea to make eye contact with the drivers waiting for the light to change. That way, you're sure they see you before you step into the crosswalk.

» **Do:** Run against traffic so you can see cars and they can see you . . . unless you're approaching a blind corner. In that case, cross the street well ahead of any cars coming toward you or from behind you to get to the safer side of the road. (See page 28 for more.)

» **Don't:** Jaywalk/run . . . unless you're in the above situation.

» **Don't:** Wear headphones . . . but if you must, keep the volume low, or one earbud out, so you can hear cars or other road users.

» **Don't:** Give drivers the bird.

» **Don't:** Wear all black or all dark colors at dusk/in the dark. It is both courteous and potentially lifesaving to wear bright colors and reflective apparel and/or safety lights.

RUNNER VS. BIKE

Look, you're both on the road to get some exercise or to get somewhere. Here's how to keep both parties happy and safe:

» **Do:** Stay out of the bike lane if there's also a sidewalk/foot-travel lane.

» **Do:** Stay far right in the bike lane if there isn't a sidewalk/foot-travel lane.

» **Do:** Give bikes the right-of-way if they're not giving it to you. It's a lot easier for you to stop and start again than it is for someone on a bike. And even if a bike *should* give you the right of way, it's better for you to yield than to get crashed into. (See "On the Trail," page 190, for more.)

» **Don't:** Wear headphones if you run in a bike lane. It's imperative to be able to hear bikes—or cyclists saying, "Excuse me," or "On the left"—when in a bike lane. Leave the headphones at home, or, if you cannot get out the door without music, wear only the right earbud so your left ear is free to hear.

RUNNER VS. DOG

Being mean to dogs on the road or trail both makes you a grump and compromises your safety. Follow these guidelines to play nicely:

» **Do:** Say things like, "Good doggie," as you pass by.

» **Don't:** Grab a dog's tail to help get you up a hill faster.

» **Do:** Give a dog (and their owner) a wide berth, if you can.

» **Don't:** Reach out to pet a dog without asking the owner first. You never know how either the dog or the owner is going to respond.

ON THE TRACK

Not having good track etiquette can make things downright uncomfortable as you're running in circles around the same people over and over. Here are some guidelines to follow:

» **Do:** Run counterclockwise (unless you get to the track and everyone is running clockwise; then, follow suit). Some locations, such as indoor tracks, might ask runners to go clockwise some days of the week and counterclockwise other days.

» **Do:** Run clockwise if you've run a lot of track lately and need to mix it up to avoid injury (see page 27). But only do this if you're the only one at the track, or if everyone else is already doing so, or if you can run in the outermost lane.

» **Do:** Take the inside lane (lane 1) while you're running intervals at your max effort.

» **Do:** Give up lane 1 to someone else who appears to be trying harder than you at that given time (and note that this does not equate that they're running faster than you), and stay in the outside lanes if you're recovering from a hard effort or walking.

» **Do:** Step off the track, or move to the outside lanes between fast efforts, if you're doing run intervals in lane 1 or 2.

» **Do:** Look over your shoulder to make sure no one's coming up fast behind you before changing lanes.

» **Do:** Stay in your lane if you're running or walking the same pace for the duration of your workout.

IN A GYM

If you're a jerk in a gym, you might be asked to leave or at least be given dirty looks. Follow these guidelines:

» **Do:** Sign up for treadmills if the gym requires you to do so.

» **Do:** Adhere to time limits on treadmills.

» **Do:** Wipe your sweat off the treadmill when you're done.

» **Don't:** Spit on the floor of the gym while running on a treadmill.

» **Don't:** Change the channel on the overhead TV without asking other gym/treadmill users if they're watching what's on, or if they mind.

» **Don't:** Conduct a business meeting on your cell phone by shouting into a headset while you're on the treadmill.

PAY ATTENTION

"Far and away, that is my number-one bit of advice," says Mark Remy, founder of DumbRunner.com and author of *The Runner's Rule Book*. "Just *pay attention*—to your own behavior, to what's happening around you, to where you are now and where you're headed. Pay particular attention to other humans, whether they're fellow runners, walkers, cyclists, or motorists. So many lapses in courtesy, civility, and even safety can be traced back to a simple lack of awareness."

ON THE TRAIL

Trails can potentially be narrow enough to only allow one trail user to pass at a time (which is why said trails are referred to as "single track"). On these types of trails, following etiquette for right-of-way becomes important for everyone's safety and enjoyment.

The general guidelines for right-of-way on the trail are that bikes should yield to runners, and runners/hikers should yield to horses. Bikes, however, have a harder time starting and stopping than do runners, so consider yielding to bikes when appropriate. Basically, whoever would have a harder time starting their momentum up again should get the right-of-way: a bike pedaling uphill, someone seemingly racing themselves, and so on. Use common sense and the golden rule to gauge right-of-way.

And if the trail is wider than a single track, stay to the right of the trail as you would on a sidewalk or shared path.

TREAD LIGHTLY

In order to preserve what makes trail environments so enjoyable, stay on designated trails. Stomping around off trail can damage delicate flora and disturb fauna. If you need to step off trail to do bodily business of any sort, choose hearty-looking ground cover (like grass) over fragile ground (like alpine flowers or moss). Release your inner naturalist.

Sucky thought zapped by this chapter:

"I don't want to make a fool of myself."

"I'm not competitive."

RACE . . . OR DON'T

Entering a race can do wonders for motivation, whether you're competitive or not. Having a race goal—like completing a 5K—can help get you out the door. Having a race goal that's different from what you usually do, like trying an obstacle or trail race if you're a (fried) seasoned road racer, can invigorate your running routine. And having paid for a race entry can add to that motivation—it can feel like you need to get your money's worth, so you'd better head on out that door and run to get ready for the upcoming race. That said, you do not have to race to call yourself a runner.

IS RACING FOR YOU? A QUIZ

If you agree with two or more of the following statements you very well might love a running-race experience:

....

1. You like parties.

....

2. You don't like parties, but you can stomach the idea of a festive atmosphere of a race where you don't have to talk to anyone if you don't want to. (A race is kind of like a moving party where some people talk and some don't.)

....

3. Your friends are afraid of you on game night (in which case, If you don't know whether you're competitive or not—you *are*).

....

4. You like testing your mettle, even if it's just against yourself.

....

5. You like the idea of being part of a parade—which a race kind of *is*—with friends or solo as people cheer you on.

....

6. You like free stuff.

....

7. You like having a goal to work toward.

....

8. You like the feeling of accomplishment.

....

WHY RACING DOESN'T SUCK

You might notice the quiz was almost guaranteed to tell you racing is for you. Here are a few reasons why signing up for a race can help you become someone who loves running:

» **Motivation.** Having a race on the calendar gets you out the door and gives your running some structure.

» **Racing is social.** You might meet potential running partners at the race. Or you could race with a bunch of friends and train for it together. And get brunch after. Mmm, brunch.

» **Racing is fun.** Whether you go easy in your race and soak up your surroundings or push yourself to see what you can do among all the other runners, the energy of a running race is contagious and fun.

» **Racing is a thrill.** It's exciting to stand in a starting corral, hear the countdown to the start of the event, hear a starting gun, and get moving with a bunch of other people. And it's exciting to cross a finish line, especially your first one.

» **Racing makes you want to get better.** No matter how you do (how you place or feel) in your first running race, you'll inevitably want to do better the next time. Running a race often starts the addicting nature of wanting to run more races and improve with each one.

» **Racing is a badge of honor.** Finishing any race of any length is an accomplishment. You might get a finisher's medal and T-shirt that will mean more to you than you think.

If none of the above appeals to you, so be it. You're still a runner even if you never run a race in your life and your runs are solely for the joy (yes, joy) of it.

HOW TO CHOOSE A FIRST RACE

Follow this order:

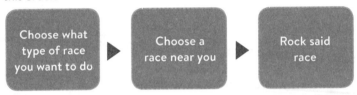

Choose what type of race you want to do ▶ Choose a race near you ▶ Rock said race

If you do decide you want to race, start small. That's not to say that no one has ever chosen a half marathon or even an ultramarathon on mountain trails as a first race, but it's advised by the gods of common sense to choose a 5K or even a mile-long race as your foray into the racing world. And if you already race and are burned out on running, consider choosing a different *type* of race from what you normally do.

WHAT TYPE OF RACE?

Picking a first race that's right for you hearkens back to knowing yourself. Though instead of taking a quiz (like you did on page 194) to figure out what kind of race is ideal for you, and specifically you, read up on the types of races that follow. Whichever one makes your heart flutter with the possibility of fun and a great sense of accomplishment but doesn't scare you so much it gives you a heart attack will be your answer.

Races of virtually any distance and on terrain ranging from flat-as-a-pancake concrete paths to climbing skyscrapers, through parks to through fire pits, exist somewhere in the world in some capacity. If you want to find the crazy ones, take to the internet. The race types listed here are the most common.

TIMED RACES OF MANAGEABLE DISTANCES:

» **1-miler.** 1 mile. Some people race hard, some people run slow, some people walk; kids can run; often held in the evening in downtown, festive environments.

» **3K.** 3 kilometers, or 1.86 miles. Some people race hard, some people run slow, some people walk; kids can run; often held in the evening in downtown, festive environments.

» **5K.** 5 kilometers, or 3.1 miles. People of all ages race hard, jog, or walk. There is no shortage of 5K races in the country, and this is a great first-race distance.[1]

UNTIMED RACES THAT PRIORITIZE FUN:

» **Mud run.** Usually 5K in distance with mud pits to crawl through and other obstacles to conquer.

» **Color run.** An untimed 5K run series where participants get doused in paint by organizers at every kilometer.

» **Bubble run.** An untimed 5K run series where participants run through colorful, sudsy bubbles every kilometer.

MORE CHALLENGING RACES THAT ARE RUNNING—PLUS OTHER STUFF:

» **Obstacle race run.** Races of varying distances, from 5K and up, where participants tackle obstacles from cargo nets, to monkey bars, to fifteen-foot walls doused in slick oil.

» **Spartan run.** Branded obstacle race, from 3 miles (and twenty obstacles) to 30 mountain miles (and sixty obstacles). Obstacles include fire, barbed wire, water, and electricity. Really.

---

1 See pages 199–200 on how to pick a race.

TIMED RACES LONGER THAN 5K:

Once you've tackled a few 5Ks, you might get the itch to add more distance. Use these races to build up to your goals and you might even discover a sweet-spot distance for yourself.

» **8K.** 8 kilometers, or 4.8 miles. A somewhat rare distance, but 8K races do exist. A common (but not sole) distance for men's collegiate cross-country races.

» **6K.** 6 kilometers, or 3.7 miles. A rare distance for a road running race, but a common (but not sole) distance for women's collegiate cross-country races.

» **10K.** 10 kilometers, or 6.2 miles. Like the 5K, 10Ks happen all the time. 10Ks sometimes have a short-distance (1K) kids' race beforehand and are sometimes run in conjunction with a 5K. Long enough to stick to your ribs, short enough that it's doable for most.

» **10-miler.** 10 miles. A great distance for easily figuring out what pace-per-mile you ran (the math is easy). Shorter, and therefore faster (if you're aiming for speed) than a half marathon. Most have frequent aid stations.

» **Half marathon.** 21.1 kilometers, or 13.1 miles. Can feel like a marathon. Frequent aid stations. A huge milestone, so to speak, for many.

» **Marathon.** 42.2 kilometers, or 26.2 miles. Fa, a long, long way to run. Most often have aid stations with water, at the least, every mile. The pinnacle for many, but completing one is absolutely not necessary to call yourself a runner.

» **Ultramarathon.** Anything longer than 26.2 miles, held on roads or trails (most are on trails). A very long way to run. Can be a great way to discover a new trail system, running (or run/walking, a method many employ, especially in the mountains) from aid station to aid station for snacks.

OFF-ROAD, TIMED RACES WITHOUT MAN-MADE OBSTACLES:

» **Trail race.** Held off road on dirt or another natural surface, often on a combination of wide path and single track. Distances range from 5K to 200 miles (yes, 200 miles at a time).

TRAIL RACE TIPS

If, on page xii, you decided that because of your nature-loving self, you would become a trail runner, and a trail running race sounds most appealing to you, great. But since a trail race is a lot different from a smooth, flat, and wide-road race, make sure you train properly leading up to the race on trails. Your body will need to get ready for the ups and downs, twists and turns, rocks, and other natural obstacles that come your way during a trail race. If you've prepped properly, a trail race can be a fantastic first race experience.

HOW TO FIND A RACE

The internet is amazing. Simply type in something like "mud run Marblehead Massachusetts," and, voilà, information for mud runs in or near Marblehead, Massachusetts, pop up in your browser. That information will include websites listing all the mud runs in that area, links to specific mud runs in that area, and places to sign up for any or all of them.

You can also learn about local races from friends and word of mouth (obvs) and by visiting your local run specialty store. Those shops are often plastered with flyers about local races, and shop employees are a knowledgeable lot who may have done some of the races they're helping to promote.

HOW TO PICK ONE OVER THE OTHER

Not all races are created equal. Factors that make some better than others include:

- fun and/or scenic courses
- good after-race parties
- good free stuff
- easy parking
- fits your budget/is worth the money

To find out if the race you're interested in fits those criteria, ask around, read race reviews online, or inquire with the race director. Another indicator of a good race is how many years it's been going on.

HOW TO SIGN UP FOR A RACE

Some races allow in-person sign-ups up until fifteen minutes before the starting gun goes off, while others sell out a year ahead of time within minutes. Research the race you're eyeing so you're ready. It's a bummer to choose and prep for a race before signing up only to find out that the race is sold out. (And if that happens to you, take your fitness and enthusiasm to another race or fun running adventure to combat the bummer.)

NOW THAT YOU'RE ALL IN . . .

Once you've chosen and signed up for a race, now what? There are goals to set (or not), there's training and preparation to be done, and then there are the race-day logistics to consider.

WALKING CAN MAKE YOU FAST!

Over his ten years as head coach to thousands of beginning runners through FastForward Sports in Boulder, Colorado, Scott Fliegelman constantly preached the benefits of alternating running and walking to his athletes. To test how well the method worked to maintain speed, he and a buddy took walk breaks in a half marathon—slowing to a walk through aid stations and letting the leaders go ahead ("Against instinct!" he says). "We found that our energy stayed remarkably steady throughout the race," he explains, "while a good number of runners ahead faded. And mentally, it really helped to break up the race into manageable chunks instead of looking at it as one long slog."

SETTING (FLEXIBLE) GOALS

You may (or may not) want to set a goal or two. When there's a race involved, it's human nature to want to set one or a few goals.

» **"A" Goal.** This goal should be slightly, just ever barely, out of reach. It should be the goal that you could achieve if every single thing perfectly falls into place: your training, the weather, your positioning in the crowd, your shoes, your apparel, your diet, your sleep, your hydration, your leg speed, your heart, your drive, your luck. An "A" goal can be a race time, a finishing place, or the goal of not walking during the race.

» **"B" Goal.** This goal should be more obtainable than your "A" goal, something like a race time or experience that you know you can accomplish thanks to your training if all things go well on race day.

» **"C" Goal.** A "C" goal is like a fallback college acceptance. You know you can get it, and you're satisfied with it, though it's okay to be disappointed that you didn't achieve your "A" or your "B" goal. A "C" goal can be something like "Don't Walk" and/or "Don't barf."

ACCEPTING YOUR RESULTS

For the sake of kindness toward yourself, productively spending your energy, and your overall mental health, do not beat yourself up if you don't achieve any of the goals you set for yourself. Maybe you didn't show up for the race or you didn't finish. Look, shit happens, and we move on.

If something—like an injury—gets in the way of being able to do the race at all, try to turn that into a positive thing. Volunteer at the race. Or use that weekend to go on a fun road trip, see a friend, or clean out a closet—you've set aside a day or weekend for the race, so do something you wouldn't normally have time to do.

KEY NO. 10 TO MAKING RUNNING NOT SUCK: PICK A FLEXIBLE GOAL

That's not to say that *flexible* means you get to a week before the race and decide you don't want to do it. *Flexible* means that if you get injured before your race, you don't force yourself to do it anyway. It also means that if you don't run your "A" or "B" goal, you won't beat yourself up over it.

HOW TO PREPARE FOR A RACE

Your running could, and likely should, change a little once you have a race on your calendar. Here are some pointers for reaching whatever goals you've set for yourself in a race, be it your first or fiftieth.

IF YOUR GOAL IS TO FINISH

If your goal race is longer than you've ever run before, and your "A" or "B" goal is to simply finish the race, you do not need to run the distance of the race before race day. Your body can do amazing things on adrenaline and make up for any mileage you didn't hit with training runs. That said, you should gradually build up to striking distance—roughly 80 percent—of the length of the race in your training. And do your final long run with enough time to recover before your race (see "What's a Taper?" page 205.)

IF YOUR GOAL IS TO RUN FARTHER AND/OR FASTER THAN EVER

If your goal for race day is to run fast at your race, you'll want to amp up your training by building up distance and speed.

» **To build up distance,** add in what's known as an "LSD" run (not as fun as it sounds). *LSD* stands for *long slow distance.* Typically, you'd do an LSD run once a week, adding time or mileage by no more than 10 percent each week to mitigate injury. For example, if the longest run you'd done to date is 2 miles, you'd increase your LSD, once-weekly run to 2.2 miles (0.2 being 10 percent more than 2 miles). Do most people adhere to *such* a gradual increase? No. But it is known to be the best way to ward off overuse injuries.

» **To build up speed,** add in one speed workout a week. On a track, warm up by jogging for five to ten minutes, then pick up the pace on the straightaways, slowing the pace back down for the curved parts of the track. You can also do a workout like this off a track. Warm up for five to ten minutes, then pick a tree or stop sign to run to, faster than your normal pace, and recover. Either way you do it, start by doing just three or four faster-than-normal-pace bursts, and always cool down. You can build up to longer stretches of "efforts" (those faster-than-normal-pace bursts) weekly.

For both LSDs and speed workouts, it's a good idea to take a day off or cross-train both the day before and the day afterward. You'll get the most out of either workout by doing it on fresh legs and you'll allow yourself to recover.

RECON

Check out the race map for the event you're signed up for and prepare for anything it might throw at you. For example, if the race climbs uphill for the first 1.5 miles, and then descends for the next 1.5 miles, it'd behoove you to do some training runs that climb and then descend. Know that you'll need to train your legs for both uphills and downs. (It's a common mistake even by seasoned runners to train for uphills but not downs. Downhills feel easy in the moment but wreak havoc on your quad muscles and your joints if you don't do them often.) And of course, if the race you signed up for has obstacles like crawling under barbed wire through a thick pit of mud or climbing up and over a slick wall by using a rope, you'll want to train your core and upper-body muscles.

TEST RUN YOUR SHOES, GEAR, FOOD, AND DRINK

Showing up to a race in a new pair of shoes or a shirt you've never worn before can ruin race day. (Blisters! Chafing!) And ingesting things on race day that you never have before during a run—like a new flavor/brand of gel at an aid station or a banana mid-run—can also ruin race day. (Poop! Barf!) If your race matters to you—and it should, since you paid for it—test run your shoes and everything else you plan on wearing on race day, down to your sunscreen and your underwear. And test run what you eat or drink both before and during your runs.

EXTRA CARE

If you ramp up your running in any way to compete in an upcoming race, you should also ramp up your self-care. That means revisiting Chapter 7 and getting out that foam roller, scheduling massages, and making sure you take rest days. It may be counterintuitive to rest more when you're training for a race, but rest days are even more important once your runs become longer and more chal-lenging. Your body needs to recover, and in order to have a successful race of any sort, you need to be able to show up to your race healthy.

HOW TO GET FASTER

Matt Fitzgerald, running coach and author of multiple running books, warns against doing training runs at race pace but says that short intervals of speed can improve times and also be a fun challenge once in a while (like once a week). "If your goal is to make progress and get better," says Fitzgerald, "throw in a hard session once in a while by warming up and then doing a handful of short—maybe thirty-second-long—sprints where you go hard but not all out. Do six of those thirty-second intervals with a minute in between. You'll notice a huge difference in your regular pace after doing runs like this once in a while."

WHAT'S A TAPER? DO I NEED TO DO IT?

Tapering is a term used to describe easing off training leading up to a race in order to be fresh and ready to go on race day. Unless you've been training your ass off by doing LSDs and speed work and want to set a PR (personal record) on race day, you do not need to taper. But if you are doing LSDs and speed work and want the best result possible at your race, then back off from running during the week or even weeks (depending on the length of your race and how much you've been training for it) leading up to it. Instead of doing the hard runs (the long or fast ones), do easy runs or take more days off than usual. And opt to cross-train (see page 125) to keep blood flowing and legs moving, instead of sitting on the couch.

RACE-DAY LOGISTICS

Race-day logistics can cause a lot of stress, but doing a little homework can help calm your nerves. You'll want to scour the race's website to find out:

- How long is the drive to the starting line?
- How early do the organizers say I need to be there?
- Where should I park?
- Do I have to pay for parking?
- Is the finish line the same place as the starting line, and if not, is there a shuttle?
- Is there food at the finish line, or should I bring something?
- Can I bring my dog? Can I push my baby in a stroller?

Answers to these types of questions can usually be found in an FAQ section on the race's website or listed elsewhere on the website.

Another race-day logistic to consider? Creating a cheering section for yourself, which can help immensely with motivation and can be fun for said cheering section. Plant friends and family along the course and at the finish line. There's nothing like looking forward to seeing a friendly face to make the miles feel shorter.

> **Tip:** If you don't intend to try to win the race, don't line up at the front at the starting line. You'll have a better experience—and you'll be practicing good etiquette—by lining up around others who may be at your same pace.

WHAT HAPPENS ON RACE DAY

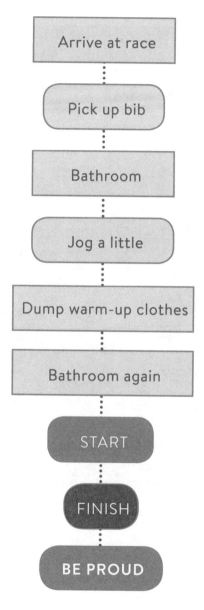

Arrive at race

Pick up bib

Bathroom

Jog a little

Dump warm-up clothes

Bathroom again

START

FINISH

BE PROUD

*If you race, be proud. The internal reward you'll have is better than any medal or race shirt.

WHAT TO BRING TO A RUNNING RACE

☐ Running shoes

☐ Running socks

☐ Running bottoms

☐ Running top

☐ Running sunglasses or hat, if using

☐ Running beanie, gloves, jacket, if using (for winter/ cold-weather races)

☐ Money

☐ Water bottle

☐ Warm-up clothes

☐ Pre-race fuel/hydration

☐ Mid-run fuel (if it'll take you forty-five minutes or longer . . . though there should be fuel on the course, so check)

☐ Post-race fuel/hydration

☐ Dry, warm clothes to change into after your race

☐ Different shoes or socks to change into after your race (if you want)

Sometimes, it's easy to stash clothes you warm up in (or stand around in) before a race back in your car before the race starts, but in some situations—like when you have to park far from the start or you took public transportation—it's a good idea to wear something you won't cry over if you lose it. Most people hanging out at races don't want to steal your old long-sleeve shirt from college that you stood around or did a warm-up jog in before the race, but wear something that you can stash in bushes by the starting line and (hopefully) grab afterward.

Sucky thought zapped by this chapter:

"Races scare me."

The Ten Keys to Making Running Not Suck

Remember, first and foremost, successful running depends on knowing yourself well and approaching running with that self-knowledge. That's the master key that unlocks all the doors. After that, there are ten individual keys that will help you get out the door, stick with it, and change your life by, basically, making running not suck.

» **Master Key: Know Thyself**

1. Visualize the New You

2. Find Your Flow

3. Run Somewhere Inspiring

4. Buy Great Gear

5. Find Your Match

6. Start Where You Are

7. Keep Your Parts Working

8. Fuel Wisely

9. Be Nice

10. Pick a Flexible Goal

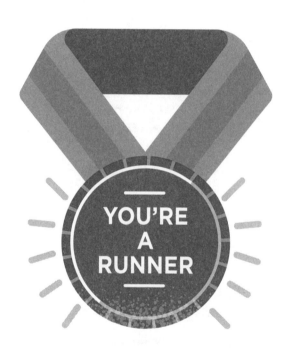

About the Author

Lisa Jhung has been running—since converting herself from initially *hating* running—for almost thirty years. She's been writing about running for almost as long. She's written for *Runner's World*, *Outside*, *Men's Journal*, *Men's Health*, and many more running-specific, women's, and general interest magazines and websites. She's the author of *Trailhead: The Dirt on All Things Trail Running* (2015).

Lisa's run everything from one-mile road races at a full sprint to triathlons and multiday adventure races. She's happiest on rambling run/walks in the woods or on beaches with her dog, with friends, or by herself. She lives in Boulder, Colorado, with her husband, Mark, and two boys, Sam and Ben, whom she regularly runs after.

Acknowledgments

This is where the author (me, Lisa) acknowledges those who helped take this book out of my head and onto paper, bound, and delivered. I'd like to thank everyone I've ever talked to about running. Why they love it, why they hate it, what about it gives them the most enjoyment (or what has kept them from loving it) . . . be it in their training, fueling, body care, racing, not racing, company, time of day, type of shoe, location, environment, et cetera. You've all inspired this book in one way or another.

I'd like to thank everyone who contributed sage, quotable advice for the book, and in particular Scott Fliegelman, Kirk Warner, Claire Shorenstein, and Charlie Merrill for going above and beyond in sharing their expertise.

Thanks to my husband, Mark, for encouraging me to write this book and for letting me run ideas by him while he cooked dinner. Thanks to my agent, Amy Elizabeth Bishop at Dystel, Goderich & Bourret LLC, for selling the idea to my awesome editor, Jess Riordan, at Running Press. Thanks to both Amy and Jess for getting my humor and letting me keep it in print, and for indulging my sometimes out-there ideas.

And thanks to Greg Straight for saving my readers from looking at my pencil sketches, and Josh McDonnell for making the whole package look pretty (and edgy and cool!).

Thanks to my published-author mother, Paula Jhung, for inspiring me to pursue the career of a free-roaming hustler (freelance writer), and my refugee father, Larry Jhung, for instilling enough strength and competitiveness in me to make that kind of life work.

I'd like to thank my sister Kelley for teaching me all the swear words and my two young sons for knowing that Mom sometimes swears (even in print!) but that it's totally not okay for them to do so. And for their general awesomeness.

INDEX

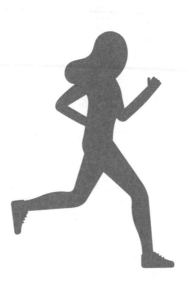